SUPERHERO
SIMPLIFIED

COLLECTED, SELECTED,
REVISED AND EXPANDED

Also by Scott Burr

SUSPEND YOUR DISBELIEF
How to Build and Build Strength with the
World's Most Rugged Suspension
Training Device

SUPERHERO SIMPLIFIED

COLLECTED, SELECTED, REVISED AND EXPANDED

SCOTT BURR

SUPERHERO
www.superherosimplified.blogspot.com
SIMPLIFIED
EST. 2013 CLEVELAND, OHIO

adp

The Artless Dodges Press
www.TheArtlessDodgesPress.com
Cleveland, Ohio

Superhero Simplified:
Collected, Selected, Revised and Expanded
Copyright © 2019 Scott Burr

ISBN-13 978-0-9907227-3-1
ISBN-10 0-9907227-3-2

Published by Superhero Simplified
www.SuperheroSimplified.blogspot.com
in partnership with
The Artless Dodges Press
www.TheArtlessDodgesPress.com
Cleveland, Ohio

Cover image from *Samson* No. 13
Pencil credit Ken Battefield
Published by Ajax-Farrell
June, 1955

Layout and cover design by The Artless Dodges Press.

CONTENTS

ABOUT THE AUTHOR

DISCLAIMER

Martial arts and/or strength training and related activities ARE DANGEROUS.

Always consult your physician before beginning any exercise program. The general information contained in this volume is not intended to diagnose any medical condition, or to replace your healthcare professional. It is advised that you consult with your healthcare professional to design an exercise program that is right for you. If you experience any pain or difficulty with any exercise, you are advised to stop and consult your healthcare provider.

The instruction and advice contained in this volume are no substitute for hands-on training with, or supervision and instruction from, an experienced and qualified professional. It is advised that before you attempt anything described or shown in this volume you consult with a qualified professional trainer. Superhero Simplified and Scott Burr disclaim all responsibility for any injury or death resulting from anything you attempt based on anything you read in this volume.

FOREWORD

Like all worthwhile pursuits, excellence is a life-long journey. And this journey is carved in stone with the discipline and relentless consistency many are not willing to endure. But it is in this great endeavor that many men, who are willing to take this journey, finally come face-to-face with their own greatness. Scott Burr is one of these men.

A master mover whose greatest strengths are yet to be uncovered, Scott has dedicated his life to the art of Jiu-Jitsu and living a life of purpose. One of life's harshest truths is the knowing that conquering one's negative self-talk and doubt is a fearless task, yet critical for any man to reach a true place of inner peace and awareness. Knowing this, Scott is not only committed to strengthening his students' minds and bodies, he also creates the spark for bringing his students to their untapped potential and their own greatness.

I am honored to call Scott Burr my friend, and appreciate all that he continues to teach me on how to be a better person, expect more of myself, and to continue my own life's work.

—Jim "Smitty" Smith
Owner, Diesel Strength & Conditioning

AUTHOR'S PREFACE

I started the Superhero Simplified blog in August, 2013. At that time I'd been running The Fight Gym—a mixed martial arts training center-turned Brazilian Jiu-Jitsu dojo and Strength & Conditioning gym—for almost six years, and I felt like I had some ideas to share.

The original concept was to give regular people (read: non-fitness professionals/athletes) practical advice and simple instruction on lifestyle, diet, fitness, martial arts, etc., and in so doing help them surprise themselves. I felt like I had finally sorted through a lot of my own misconceptions about training, and could see where other people were struggling.

I stopped posting new content on the Superhero Simplified blog in 2016. I felt that my overall perspective on martial arts and physical fitness had evolved, and I wanted a new venue whose tone reflected the change. That effort, however—www.JiuJitsuDoMaeda.com—never grew into much beyond a few blog posts. I have included those posts in this volume, along with some materials that I prepared for private clients during this same time period. I have also included essays and excerpts that I wrote in the years since, but have not published.

When it comes to posts relating to fitness and physical conditioning, I have retained pieces where I felt the content might offer some food for thought to readers for whom fitness and working out are already a fact of life. I have, however, left out content where I simply describe a workout or a protocol. These pieces will be compiled into a later volume.

The contents of this book have been proofread for errors and selected for relevance, but except where noted they have not been edited for content or updated to reflect my current thoughts or training methods. That being said, I have not included here anything that I no longer feel to be fundamentally sound.

These materials represent a distinct era in my own martial arts and fitness journey, and compiling them into this volume has given me the opportunity to reconnect with that time. It is not often that you're given the chance to look at the world through your younger self's eyes. It has been an interesting and often illuminating experience, and I am grateful to have had the chance.

As always, it is my hope that what I have written here will help you discover or rediscover just how much potential you have, and just how super you can be.

I wish you all nothing but the best that life has to offer.

Scott Burr
Cleveland, Ohio
May 11, 2019

START HERE

Originally published on SuperheroSimplified.blogspot.com
August 27, 2013

Welcome to Superhero Simplified!

My name is Scott Burr. I'm a Brazilian Jiu-Jitsu instructor and Strength & Conditioning coach. I run a training facility called The Fight Gym located in Chagrin Falls, Ohio. Over the years I've developed, adopted, borrowed and co-opted a wide array of training methods, training philosophies, diet plans, and equipment designs; I've tinkered and created, refined, and redesigned my methods and my tools, always looking for new ways to achieve the best results for myself and my students and clients. This blog is a place for me to collect these ideas and share them with any like-minded individuals out there.

Why the name Superhero Simplified? Because when I was a little kid, I wanted to be Batman.

No: I really, *really* wanted to be Batman. How bad? I could tell you about the time I jumped off the porch wearing a set of collapsable hang-glider wings I'd fashioned out of wood scraps and garbage bags. Or I could describe the time I swung off the tree in our backyard with a rope tied to my "utility belt." I could recite any of a number of incidents that took years off my mother's life, but maybe it's better if you just believe me when I say that I really, really wanted to be the Caped Crusader.

Then, like all little boys, I grew up. I went off to college, studied English Literature, and bounced around out West. I studied martial arts (first the Korean style Kuk Sul Do, then Muay Thai, Boxing, American Freestyle Wrestling, and Gracie Jiu-Jitsu), spent a good deal of time rock climbing, and eventually settled back in the small Midwestern town where I was born and raised.

When I turned thirty, as people do when these milestone birthdays come around, I took stock. Like everyone else who has ever walked the planet, my life's story was a mixed bag of successes and disappointments. On the one hand, I wasn't the bestselling novelist I thought I would be. On the other hand, I was nearing the rank of black belt in Gracie Jiu-Jitsu and, as I was (and still am) working as a GJJ instructor, this was a big part of my life and personal point of pride. I wasn't living the life of the "climber bum," following the seasons from Southern California to Yosemite, but I had helped to build a unique martial arts and strength & conditioning facility, and in the process had become part of a community.

Looking back it occurred to me that, while my stated goals had evolved with my age, my various pursuits had actually moved me toward another, earlier goal. I'd learned to fight, to ascend and descend fantastic heights, to condition my body and challenge my mind. Wasn't this the mold of the comic book hero I'd most emulated as a child? What was my life, if not an adult's expression of a child's wish to be the Dark Knight?

This blog is meant to be a resource for any and everyone looking to change their diet, increase their fitness level, learn an awesome skill (How to choke a bad guy unconscious! How to rig a rappel!), and basically become a superhero. Will I teach you how to leap tall buildings in a single bound? No, but I will show you the methods I've used to maintain and increase my health, fitness, and competence.

So what are you waiting for? It's time to be super!

MEN SEEKING FAILURE

Originally published on SuperheroSimplified.blogspot.com
September 13, 2013

Take a second to think this through with me.

If you come to the gym and work out with me, and at the end of the workout I'm beat and talking about how hard it was, and you say something like, "It wasn't really that bad," or, "the only really hard part was ____," to what do you attribute this discrepancy?

There are two options, right? Either 1) you're stronger/tougher/in better shape than me, or 2) you and I did different workouts.

Logically it must be #1, right? Because you know that we did the same workout, right? But do you really think that's the case? Really?

I'm not trying to claim that I'm the toughest, fittest guy on the planet. I am trying to say that if 1) you think I'm fitter/stronger/tougher than you, and 2) you work out with me and I have a harder time than you do, the discrepancy probably lies in what you're doing. And it might hold the key to why you're not seeing the kind of results you want to be seeing.

Before I go any further, then, I have to ask the question: What is the purpose of exercise? What does it do? Why should I do it? What am I doing to myself or for myself when I go into the gym?

11

The answer is that exercise conditions your body to greater stress —mechanical, cardiovascular, etc.—than it was previously acclimated to. It's not a great tool for weight loss when compared to diet change, and cosmetic alteration is more dramatically and more effectively achieved through body fat loss (via diet change) than through exercise. Further, the extreme stress of a prolonged high intensity workout cannot in and of itself be called "healthy." (Is throwing yourself down a flight of stairs or running from an angry dog healthy? This is the kind of stress/damage you are subjecting yourself to.)

So let me ask you: Do you have this purpose in mind when you come to the gym? Do you go in with the intention of challenging yourself, or do you go in with some vague notion that exercise is "good" for you, or that you're going to work off the six beers and the chocolate cake you had last night? (News flash: you're not.)

Play a quick little mind game with me. I'll make a statement, and you rebut.

I am not physically able to do twenty-five strict push-ups. I fail around fifteen.

You can't do twenty-five, either. I bet you fail sooner than I do.

What did your brain just do? Did it say, "Wait a minute, Scott doesn't even know me!" Did it say, "This cocky, know-it-all, so-and-so." Did it say, "I can totally do twenty-five push-ups! I'll do them right now!" Did it say, "I must have been wrong, thinking Scott was strong/tough/handsome/a worthwhile coach/trainer/fighter."

Or did you say: "Jesus Christ, what do those push-ups look like? Show me those!"

So let me go back and say, I can do twenty-five "push-ups." Hell, I can do fifty. So can you, I'm sure. But I don't care (and you shouldn't care, either) about the push-ups that I (or you) can do fifty reps of. I care (and you should care) about the ones that make me (and you) fail at fifteen.

If you come to a workout thinking of it as a test of your physical ability then the tendency is for you to do the versions of the exercises that you are already able to do. If I tell you to do ten push-ups and you see that as a test (is "I," the entity, capable of overcoming this challenge?) then you are emotionally invested in the outcome (I don't want to fail! If I fail it reflects poorly on me/diminishes me/affects the way I see myself and the way others see me!) and you have a strong emotional incentive to perform those push-ups in a manageable way, so that you can pat yourself on the back at the end and think better of "I" ("I" did it! "I" am capable! "I" am as strong as Scott! Scott's challenge was no match for "I"!).

My question to you is: WHAT IN THE HELL IS THE POINT OF THAT?!?! You came to the gym to work out, which means that you came to the gym to condition your body to greater stress than it was previously acclimated to, which means you came to the gym to FAIL. If you do the push-ups you can already do then WHY WOULD YOUR BODY ADAPT? It was already capable of doing those ten garbage push-ups!

This is not about you and me. This is not about which of us is stronger or fitter or better looking. This is and always was about YOU and YOU. Good for you that you don't think the workout was very hard. Six months of your half-assed version of my workout is going to leave you exactly where you were six months ago.

Really think about this for a second. You are not wasting my time or energy when you do those wide grip, partial range of motion push-ups: YOU ARE WASTING YOUR TIME AND ENERGY. The emotional bolster you gain by "beating" my workouts isn't worth one iota of actual improvement.

I want you to be strong. I want you to be superhero, mutant, animal strong. But the borderland between what I can do for you and what you have to do for yourself is forever your domain. I can tell you that push-ups follow squats, I can challenge you to a certain extent, but I can't make you challenge yourself. If you come in looking to bolster your ego by overcoming "tests" then you are interested in what you ARE, not what you're trying to become. And that, frankly, is a stupid, stupid waste.

Don't come into the gym afraid of failing. Come into the gym seeking failure.

See you on the mats.

I CAN MOVE THINGS WITH MY MIND

Originally published on SuperheroSimplified.blogspot.com
September 16, 2013

My name is Scott, I run the Superhero Simplified blog, and I can move things with my mind.

No, seriously. I can move things, even heavy things. I can lift them up, I can move them around, I can set them down somewhere else.

I can even move myself.

In fact, this fantastic power is what I'm using to type these words right now.

All right, you caught me. When I say I can move things with my mind—that I can lift them up and move them around—I mean that I can direct my body to lift things up and move them around. When I say that I'm using this power to type this post, I mean that my brain is telling my fingers how to move, and which keys to push.

And yeah, I know that was an obnoxious gimmick. But before you stop reading, take one second to really think about this basic but no less incredible ability. Think—really think—about what it means to have a body that is at your brain's command.

One of my favorite maxims at The Fight Gym is: Your body is a tool for turning intention into effect. You want something from the next room, you walk into the next room and pick it up. You need a shelf in your bedroom, you build a shelf. You want better health, greater flexibility, more strength, you do the things you need to do to produce those effects.

Really think about that. Your body is the interface between your brain and its intangible musings and the tangible world in which you live: the interface through which your *immaterial* thoughts may become *material* reality.

More than this, your body is a tool capable of *modifying* its ability and effectiveness. As in: two days ago I could lift ten pounds, yesterday I made myself lift ten pounds ten times, now I can lift twelve pounds. (Or, conversely: Yesterday I ate Skittles for breakfast, lunch, and dinner, and today I'm bloated, my joints hurt, and I feel like I'm getting a cold.)

So you say: So what? I already know this. Everybody knows this, and it isn't anything even remotely like a super power.

To you I say: Isn't it?

Have you ever watched a very young child playing with an object, throwing it away and picking it up and throwing it away again? Can you recall or imagine that hypnotic fascination that *I*, this form, have caused this other *thing*—not a part of myself but wholly exterior, wholly *other*—to move, to fall, to fly: that I have enacted this change upon my surroundings?

I know, I know: this is extremely basic. But this is exactly why it is so important that we stop and consider it. This physical existence, this strange manifestation of some cosmic compulsion toward collection and adhesion, toward atomic bonding and gravitational attraction, this solid reality is malleable by me.

When we remember this, we suddenly rediscover that child's fascination: that this basic ability—which most of us take for granted at every waking moment of every day—is, in fact, an incredible thing.

But, you say, why bother writing a post about it? If it's so basic as to be absolutely inextricable from our daily existence (if you got

16

out of bed this morning, if your brain told your body to sit up and walk, you've already used it) then why do we need to say anything about it?

The answer to that question can be summed up in one word: disembodiment.

People talk to me. When we get past the introductions and into the, "What do you do for a living?" phase of the conversation, and I tell them I run a gym, they start talking. "I've got to get in better shape," they say. "I used to run/play tennis/bike/lift weights, but in these past couple years I've gotten away from it." They say, "I know I need to get back into it, but it's hard with everything I've got going on." They say, "It's hard to find/keep the motivation."

They say, "I know I could stand to lose ten/fifteen/thirty/forty pounds." They say, "I know I need to eat better." They say, "I really like beer." They say, "It's Thanksgiving/Christmas/a birthday party. You've got to have pumpkin pie/cookies/cake." They say, "I mean, I think I'm generally pretty healthy."

To me, these statements are symptoms of a basic problem endemic in modern America. As we become increasingly technology focused (on both the production and consumption ends), as we are increasingly told that "it's what's on the inside that counts," as food industry concerns bombard us with advertisements for their products such that our dietary common sense is drowned out (here's a diet tip for anyone looking for one: eat only foods with one ingredient), as proxy experience becomes more effective/fulfilling (video games supplant the excitement of real experience, online communities assuage the yearning for actual contact, movies and TV shows allow us to vicariously experience travel, adventure, etc.) we live more and more from the neck up, disconnected from everything south of the collar bones, and we find ourselves in a strange moment where the body has become a mystery to its inhabitant: he becomes fat or sick or weak and doesn't understand how it happened.

"I wasn't doing anything too bad!" he says. "I wasn't doing anything that everybody else wasn't also doing!"

But of course that's the problem: American normal is pretty messed up. And the fact of the matter is that if you participate in American normal—if you watch your 34 hours of TV a week (that's the average) and you drink your 78 liters of beer and eat your 100 pounds of refined sugar a year (both average) then you're going to experience some negative health effects.

I in no way mean to disparage technology or progress or America. I do want to remind everyone, however, that—as Joe Frazier famously said—if you kill the body, the head will die. You are not just a personality living in a body—you *are* the body. One is inextricable from the other.

So my point to you is this: Don't take your body and all of its amazing abilities for granted. You are the owner of a marvelous machine that responds to your every command: Don't just use it to type "facebook.com" into the navigation bar. Don't just use it to change the channel, or put chicken nuggets in your mouth. Don't just use it to move a pen to fill in forms at a job you hate. Respect it, cherish it, and maintain it.

Then recognize that the world is your canvas, and your body is your brush. Shouldn't you paint something? This can mean pushing yourself to lift more weight or run a four minute mile, but it can also even mean pruning a tree or changing the laces on your shoes or building a shelf or moving a dresser. It can mean doing anything that reminds you that you are capable, and maybe even powerful. And maybe—just maybe—even super.

LIVE FREE OR DIET

Originally published on SuperheroSimplified.blogspot.com
September 23, 2013

I've been involved in martial arts and fitness for almost fifteen years, but it's only in more recent years that I've begun to seriously consider my diet as an important component of both my training and my overall health.

Part of this is age. I started in the martial arts when I was seventeen, a high school kid, and though I was never quite as lean as I wanted to be, I was content (or content enough not to seriously examine the issue) to shrug this off as poor genetics. I figured I just had one of those body types that stored more subcutaneous fat, and I didn't believe that anything I did was going to make much of a difference: after all, I was training martial arts all the time, biking five miles up and down hills to and from class; I was doing everything right, as far as I understood it, and I could only conclude that the body I had, after all that effort, was the best body I was going to get.

Through the end of my teens and my early and mid-twenties, "diet" remained an afterthought. I tried out various notions here and there for a few weeks or a few months at a time—low or no fat, no eating after six p.m., fasting from noon until the following morning, high protein, high carb, etc. The rest of the time, when I wasn't on one of these kicks, I ate pretty much whatever I wanted: I never noticed a difference in how I looked or felt anyway, so what did it matter? Nothing I was going to do was going to change the body I was stuck with: what I had, experience was teaching me, was the best I could hope for.

It's hard for me to nail down exactly when my thinking changed, or why, but a few key events stand out. When I was twenty-six I spent an entire summer plagued by oppressive fatigue and the feeling that I was "drifting." It was a bit like vertigo: I felt like my head was a boat that had come untied from its dock (my body) and was starting to gradually float away. I went to the doctor and explained my symptoms.

"What do you do for work?" he asked me.

"I teach mixed martial arts," I said.

"I think you may be overtraining," he said.

"Yeah?" I said, with what I'm now sure was an obvious mix of pride and skepticism in my voice: overtraining was just what the weak and the wimpy called training hard, wasn't it?

"Describe your average week of training to me," he said.

"Sure," I said, and launched into a description of Monday's training, which at that time consisted of Brazilian Jiu-Jitsu in the morning, an hour of high-intensity interval training in the afternoon, and three hours of classes in the evening. I was getting ready to describe Tuesday when he cut me off.

"Yeah," he said, "you're overtraining."

They drew some blood and sent the sample off to the lab—"Just to make sure there's nothing else going on"—and I left there feeling like I always felt leaving the doctor's office: like they couldn't tell me anything, like I shouldn't have bothered, like doctors all want their patients to sit in sterilized, padded rooms all day to eliminate every opportunity for illness or injury. I went back to training at breakneck pace, and I figured the fatigue and the vertigo would pass, sooner or later, and I didn't think any more about the doctor until his office called to let me know that my results were back, and that my white blood cell count was way, way down: that I really needed to pump the brakes a bit.

I backed off, but not much. I was full of that particular brand of pride that is really just fear in disguise: fear that the tenuous gains I'd made, the fitness level I'd achieved, the things about myself and my body that I liked would disappear if I let up on the throttle. Other people, the thinking went, had won the genetic lottery: they had the luxury of low body fat and good muscle tone; I had to work for every crease and ripple, had to pound the pavement and beat my body into submission.

Again, I chalk a lot of this up to my age. I was twenty-six, and I still thought in an abstract way that my experience or physiology or psychology was innately different from everyone else's. Running helped other people get lean; it didn't work like that for me. High-carb, low-fat diets helped other people lose weight; I didn't see much of a difference. Other people wanted to quit after six rounds of heavy sparring; I would go the seventh and eighth. Other people didn't have the discipline to get into the gym every day; I did. Other people saw the world one way; I saw it another way. Other people were content to work a nine-to-five and pursue the American Dream; I wasn't. Looking back, I see this for what it is: the juvenile egotism of someone whose self-worth is tied up in his "artistic disposition," the fallacious belief of a young man whose worldview is so warped that he gleans emotional affirmation and nourishment from his self-aggrandized isolation.

Again, I'm not sure exactly when things changed. The longer I went the more tired I became, and the less nourished I felt by my perception of myself (as a vaguely self-destructive hard-charger) and others' perception of same (someone saying, "You're insane," to me regarding one of my workouts had once fueled me for hours). Practically, my priorities changed: I wasn't fighting anymore, and I was feeling less and less at home in the increasingly-meathead world of Mixed Martial Arts, both as a trainer and a fan. I still loved Brazilian Jiu-Jitsu, and I still loved the capabilities my fitness level afforded me both on and off the mat, but I was questioning my methods and my outlook. Was all of this training really good for me? What was the difference between the kind of damage I did to myself in a hard workout and the kind of damage someone might do to themselves at a bar on a Friday night? What did my supposed "fitness" matter, when I felt too stiff and sore and tired to get out of bed some mornings? What did it matter, if my white blood cell count was notably diminished by these actions? Wasn't I, in effect, making myself *less* healthy, less fit?

These questions arose in conjunction with certain minor but no less acute symptoms (though "symptoms" almost feels like too strong a word here) that I began experiencing. Wheat (bread, beer, pasta) started making me profoundly tired. Like: "It's been nice seeing you, but now I have to go home" tired. Corn upset my stomach and left a bad taste in my mouth. Sugary foods started making me crash super hard. I don't know whether this feedback had been there all along and I'd just been ignoring it, or if it became more pronounced as I approached thirty, but once I tuned in, there was no tuning back out. Food—the thing that was supposed to nourish me and give me energy—was seemingly doing the opposite.

So, to review: training, the thing that was supposed to make me fit, was making me less fit. Food, which was supposed to fuel me and keep me healthy, was seemingly a drag on my system. Clearly something was wrong on a basic, systemic level. Training was my job, my passion, my life, and I was going about it wrong. All of the energy I had poured into it and was still pouring into it had brought me here: exhausted and broken down, but still chained to a mill wheel that I had to keep pushing for fear of what I would lose if I stopped.

22

The process that followed is ongoing, and has led me to reevaluate many (if not most, if not all) of my assumptions about health and fitness. Despite my years of implementation, I found on closer inspection that many of my notions about diet and exercise were founded on nothing more than weight room chatter, advice from school sports coaches (most of these were parents or teachers paid a part-time salary to coach a sport, with no background in physical education or training), magazine articles, television programs, and even food labels (how often have you let your dinner tell you that it's healthy? I.e. The box says no fat; that must be a good thing, if they're advertising it!). But now the trial was over and the jury was back: these ideas didn't work, or didn't work very well. I had used them all, and they hadn't delivered on their promises.

Worse, when nudged in the right direction, the answer was obvious. I didn't need to eat a special diet made up of engineered food: I needed to eat real food, and eat it exclusively. I didn't need to smash my body into submission: I needed to prompt it to adapt with intelligent provocation, and then give it the time it needed to recover. There was no mystery: health and fitness weren't an elusive pot of gold at the end of some grueling rainbow; they were my body's natural state, a state which every second of every hour of every day my self-replicating cells were working diligently to achieve. All I had to do was get out of their way, and not inhibit them with my behavior or my diet. Health was what felt good: not the false pleasure of a sugar high but the sustainable and stable energy of real nourishment; not the swaggering self-satisfaction of a vomit-inducing workout, but the supple comfort of a strong and efficient and functional body.

Let me be clear: most weeks I still train seven days. But my hard workouts are fewer and farther between: instead of sparring, conditioning, extra conditioning, and marathon cardio sessions, now I do specified high-intensity interval training twice a week, for no more than 45 minutes total each session, and that time includes rest. I train BJJ pretty much every day, but with the exception of a few rolls here and there this training is light and playful. I have noticeably less body fat than I did when I was training my hardest, and am significantly stronger. (I don't have any numbers here, so you'll just have to believe me.) The most important thing, though, is how much better I feel. I'm not tired all the time. I've lost the floaty, vertigo feeling. My digestion is easy (I don't have bloating or an upset stomach, both of which were common issues in the past). Since changing my diet and training I haven't had a cold or been sick. Even my seasonal allergies—a mainstay of my life up to this point—have significantly abated.

As I've said, I spent several years training with the same ineffective methods partially out of fear that, should I stop, I would lose what ground I had gained against what I thought then was my body's inherent unfit state. This aspect, this stubbornness, I can understand, but I wonder why I didn't change my diet sooner. After all, I did know better. I knew that frozen pizza wasn't the fuel my body wanted. I knew that beer wasn't helping me get stronger. The hangovers—both food- and alcohol-induced—were pretty clear indicators that something wasn't working. So why didn't I listen? Why didn't I change my diet then?

I think about this whenever someone asks me about my diet, and I watch their eyes glaze over a minute into my response. I think they must be feeling what I felt back then: that the task of "dieting"—of being ever-vigilant against temptation and misstep—is a monumental, confining, and after all, probably not-all-that-rewarding endeavor. ("It doesn't matter what I eat or don't eat," I used to think, "I'm always going to look about the same; I'm never going to be as cut as I want to be.") "That's all well and good," they think, "but I have to live in the world, and I love food, and what if it's my birthday and someone makes a cake, or what if it's Thanksgiving and there's pumpkin pie, or Halloween and there's candy, etc., etc."

It seems to me that most people think of dieting in this way: that they can either live free, enjoying the whole smorgasbord of life, or they can be reserved and austere and thin, enjoying their plain water and celery sticks. The word "diet" itself has come to connote this kind of self-restriction: "I'm going on a diet," someone says, and immediately we think of self-denial, of pleasures forsaken, of an unpleasant (but thankfully short-term) sojourn in the land of tasteless "health food" and un-indulged cravings.

If I could only give you one piece of health advice, it would be to take this definition and throw it away. Despite what the word has come to signify in recent years, "diet" first and foremost refers to the food—good, bad, or indifferent—that a person eats. You have a diet, right now, and every day you compose this diet. You go to the cupboard or the refrigerator and you pull something out and you put it in your mouth. This is not simply something that happens, like the sun rising or your heart beating. That food does not go into you until you put it there, and the question you have to ask yourself is: What is your diet doing for you? Because your diet doesn't just happen: *You make it happen.*

Eating healthier foods isn't about not eating unhealthy food, it's about eating healthy food on purpose. It's not a negation: It's an intentional act in pursuit of nourishment. Because that is the purpose of eating: your body needs raw materials to do the work it's doing all the time, every day, building you into a vital, strong, resilient, healthy you.

If the change in my diet was simply about weight loss, I would have quit by now. Despite its seemingly paramount importance in our society, having a flat stomach is hard to enjoy: certainly you have moments of pride standing in front of the mirror, or when someone compliments your appearance, but these are fleeting when compared to the immediate sensory pleasure of chocolate cake or pizza, fresh from the oven. It is not my love of my appearance that keeps me comfortably "on track," but the tangible sensory pleasure of feeling good. I don't want the chocolate cake not because I'm so worried about waking up flabby tomorrow, but because I really understand how lousy it will make me feel, as soon as the initial buzz wears off.

People ask me if I have trouble not eating bread and my answer is, "No, but I have no trouble not eating broken glass, either." I have no trouble not putting something into my body that I know will make me feel worse.

A good diet, a bad diet, a liquid diet, a fruit diet, a college diet—none of it just happens. Each one is intentionally created day by day, minute by minute, forkful by forkful. I encourage you to eat on purpose: to think about what your food (which you bought and paid for, after all, with money you expended effort to earn) is doing for you. If you do that, you'll be well on your way to superhero status.

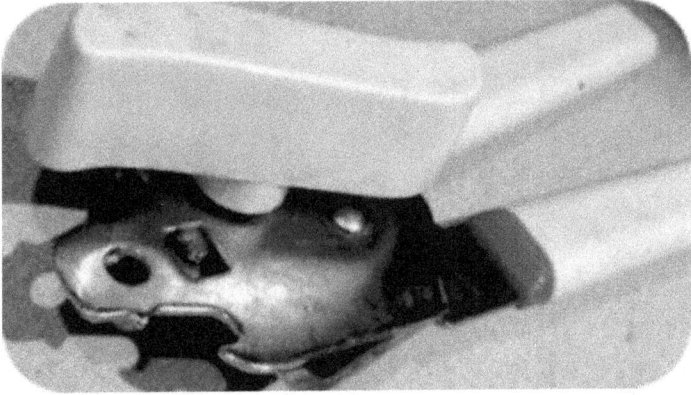

CAN OPENER

Originally published on SuperheroSimplified.blogspot.com
September 30, 2013

This is our can opener.

We've had this can opener for years, and for years I've been saying, "We've got to get a new can opener," because this can opener never, ever worked right.

Get out a can, everything's going great. Get out the opener, everything is still on track. Clamp the jaws down tight, so that the disk breaks through the lid, and we're off to the races. Start turning the handle, and the wheels come off the whole endeavor. Every time, without fail, the turning disk—the component responsible for moving the can around in a neat little circle—walks the can's lip free of the opener's mechanism, and what was once a happy and functional union becomes instead a comedy of errors. A half dozen tries later and you're lucky if these abortive efforts add up to a majority circumference, lucky if the vicious and jagged edges of your ill-fated attempts don't leave you bleeding into your Spaghetti-Os.

"That's it," I would say. "The next time we go to Bed, Bath, & Beyond we're getting a new can opener."

—

People are funny creatures. It's hard to imagine a lion or an aardvark or a squirrel doing something ineffective over and over again. The forces of evolution have weeded out the adherents to any ineffective method (after all, these significantly diminish survival potential) and what's left are furry geniuses: critters who are brilliant at executing their specific survival skills. The lion knows how to stalk the gazelle; the otter knows how to crack open the clam. As humans, we're obviously pretty good at surviving too, but for most of us (for you, if you're reading this on a computer screen) the forces of evolution bear down less acutely. After all: I'm probably not going to starve to death if I can't get my stupid can opener to work. A comfortable buffer exists between us and the necessity of a survival imperative, and this is where we seem to get in our own way.

Self-consciousness can be a blessing and a curse. The ability to imagine a theoretical self experiencing possible outcomes to an action, and then avoid those involving injury or death in real life, is arguably the reason we're still on this planet. The ability to imagine yourself as something that you're not —fitter, stronger, more successful, etc.—is the root of human aspiration. But (as any middle-schooler will tell you) self-consciousness can also be a heavy, stifling burden. And, as anyone suffering from anxiety or social phobias will attest, self-consciousness can very quickly become a prison.

For most of us, though, in our day-to-day lives, self-consciousness is neither of these extremes. Most of us don't spend our days making life-or-death decisions, nor do we spend them paralyzed by self-examination. Most of the time, this fantastic capacity is relegated to more mundane tasks. "I'm hungry," we think. "What do I have in the refrigerator?" We imagine ourselves going to the refrigerator and having a look, or maybe we remember the last time we went shopping. We remember that we have meat and lettuce and cheese and we think, "Maybe I'll make tacos." We imagine ourselves eating the tacos, and we feel an echo of the visceral pleasure of the taste and texture and smell. We decide that, Yes, we will make tacos. But we're out of salsa. We imagine going to the store, how long it will take...

—

Those of you involved in self-defense training or combat sports may already be familiar with the concept of the O.O.D.A. loop. For those of you who aren't familiar: the concept was developed by USAF Colonel John Boyd, and describes the four-step process that the human brain goes through when presented with stimuli. Simply put: whenever any of us is presented with a situation we 1) Observe the situation, 2) draw upon our training, preconceived notions, cultural tradition, etc. to Orient ourselves to the salient details of that situation, 3) Decide what to do about the salient details, and 4) Act upon that decision.

The O.O.D.A. loop concept comes up a lot in the context of military and police training, and accordingly it is easy to forget its broader application. The fact is, the loop is running all the time, processing everything you see and encounter. Yes, it's running when you step out into the street and a car is suddenly coming at you, but it's also running when you need to open a can of chicken broth and all you've got to use is the stupid can opener you've been meaning to replace for years.

Because your O.O.D.A. loop relies on your ability to identify salient details and orient to those details, your O.O.D.A. loop is always at the mercy of your ability to effectively and accurately discern the significance of what you observe. The failure of this capacity is often big news—police shoot an unarmed suspect, misidentifying a wallet as a gun—but it can also lay the groundwork for more mundane failures.

Because the fact of the matter is: There is nothing wrong with my can opener. There was something wrong with the way I was using it.

For some reason I had it stuck in my head that the opener, when engaged, should stand in line with the side of the can, and despite the opener's tendency toward its proper angle I would always force it straight, favoring my inaccurate vision of "proper use" even in the face of ongoing failure. It was only when I stopped thinking I "knew" how the can opener was supposed to work, and let it work on its own, that I got the lid off the can on the very first try.

—

There's a much longer blog post in here somewhere, about ego and our tendency to defend a decision even in the face of overwhelming dissenting evidence. For now though, I want to make a more modest point. I've noticed a tendency among some martial artists and fitness enthusiasts toward what I call the formula approach: "If I do X sets of Y exercises on odd-numbered days," they say, "and A sets of B exercises on even-numbered days, I'll get the body I want." Or, "If I roll three days a week and watch instructional videos on YouTube for an hour a night, I'll get better/get my next belt/tap the toughest guy in the room." This sort of intentional, regimented goal-setting is absolutely commendable and is inarguably the path toward definite progress. It is, however, important to remember that these regimens are created using the best information you have at the time. You are orienting to the situation with the information you have gleaned from experience and training up to that point. If six months down the road you haven't reached your goal, or you've only made it part of the way, it is essential that you take that new information into consideration and re-orient. I've seen too many people married to fitness or diet plans that aren't producing the promised results, running mile after mile in the Cleveland winters or pounding away on a treadmill, eating endless bowls of pasta because a vegetarian diet is supposed to help them lose weight. Goals are important and discipline is essential, but you don't earn any points for blindly adhering to a dogma that is not serving you.

So I say to you: remember the story of Super Scott, and the broken can opener that wasn't really broken. Observe, Orient, Decide, and Act, but don't be afraid to Observe the result and RE-orient. Your time is precious and always running out: don't waste it riding buses that aren't taking you where you're trying to go. Do that, and I'm sure you'll have no problem staying super.

SELF-MOTIVATED SAM, AND HOW HE'S BEEN LIED TO

Originally published on SuperheroSimplified.blogspot.com
October 7, 2013

My grandmother used to tell me that her son, my uncle, was "into that same exercising that you do."

My Uncle Bob follows the "weights and cardio" model of physical fitness. I favor high-intensity interval training and sport-specific drilling.

To me, the difference is obvious. To my grandmother, of course, there was no difference. To her, my uncle and I were both just "into exercising."

My grandparents grew up during the Depression. Later, my grandfather ran a tool and die shop in Syracuse, New York. To their generation, going to work more often than not meant going to *work*. Jobs typically involved at least some manual labor, and everything from mowing the lawn to putting up the storm windows demanded physical engagement. It wasn't necessary to set aside a special time during the day to be intentionally physical, and the very suggestion would have sounded absurd to my grandparents and just about everyone they knew.

Of course, a lot has changed since my grandparents' day. Our economy is increasingly soft-skill and tech-skill based, and our lives are increasingly lived digitally and online, and as a result many of us live unhealthily sedentary lives. Accordingly, we are experiencing what some authorities have dubbed "an obesity epidemic." According to the Centers for Disease Control, more than one-third of adults in the United States are obese, and obesity-related conditions (heart disease, stroke, and type 2 diabetes) are among the nation's leading causes of preventable death. While this is troubling, it should be noted that this epidemic has resulted in counter efforts on the part of various groups, corporations, and government bodies to highlight the importance of physical activity. A few generations ago, "working out" was a strange concept: now it seems that everyone I talk to takes it for granted that exercise is good for them. "I need to start running again," they say. Or, "I need to get back in the gym." The average person can probably even tell you some basic "facts" about different types of exercise: do cardio to lose fat, lift weights to get big, etc. This is all a far cry from my grandparents' day, when the idea that exercise was an important component of health was far from the norm.

Our bodies are incredibly resilient, but then again they have to be: they are also incredibly breakable. Exercise, by definition, asks more of your body than might otherwise be asked: you are putting your body under physical strain to prompt a stress response, whether that means red blood cell production or muscle tissue repair. Asking more of your body can be productive or, if you take it too far, it can be disastrous, and with that in mind I think it's worth taking a second look at what a lot of us do in the name of "health."

We have arrived at a strange moment culturally, where people are encouraged to work out and bombarded with advice, much of it incomplete or misguided, and then often left to their own devices. For most people this situation is fairly harmless: the average person isn't going to do anything intensely enough to injure themselves and for most people, the low-intensity intermittent "something" is far better than the "nothing" they would likely do otherwise. But for the disciplined and dedicated, for those whose constitutions compel them to exercise—to wake up early and pound the pavement, to hit the gym even after a long and stressful and tiring day—these misguiding moments can lead to frustration, plateaus, and even injury.

Let's take my friend, Self-Motivated Sam.

Sam is motivated and driven. Sam makes fitness a priority. Sam "knows" what everyone in America "knows": that running is the best exercise for building cardiovascular endurance. That long-phase cardio is the best way to lose body fat. That high reps with light weight tones muscles, while low reps with heavy weight builds muscles. Sam knows that eating fat makes you fat, and that the key to being lean is a low-fat diet. Sam can't tell you how he knows these things: they're things that everyone knows. They're pieces of information that float around the weight room at school, or that coaches pass along, or that he reads in health magazine articles. He knows these things because his roommate told him, or because a brand of granola bar produced a lower-fat version of its product with the tagline that it was the "healthier choice."

Sam takes these pieces of information and he forms a plan for himself. He dedicates hours and hours over years and years to the plan he has outlined. He sweats and bleeds and expends his energy. When he doesn't see the results he wants, when he begins to burn out, he chastises himself for his lack of commitment, or tells himself that he's been slacking, and he rededicates himself to his plan. Maybe he needs to run five times a week instead of three. Maybe he needs to lift heavier weights. Maybe he needs to cut out fat entirely.

The Self-Motivated Sams of the world are the ones who suffer at the hands of what has now become "common knowledge." They're the ones who repeat the behavior long enough for the flaws in the system to manifest, for the risks to play out. Typically it's the Sams who have hip replacements at 40, who sustain life-altering injuries (chronic or acute), who eventually collapse into a jumble of arthritis and chronic inflammation. "I used to be in really good shape," they say. "I used to run and lift and bike and swim." They never seem to ask the question: If I was in such "good shape," if I was so "healthy," then why did my body disintegrate? Why am I in worse shape now than the people who exercised intermittently through their 20s and 30s and 40s?

For a long time, I was Sam. As I've discussed in previous posts, I followed "conventional wisdom" as far as it would take me, and found that it didn't lead where I wanted to go, or where it promised that it would. My performance was suffering, my immune system was suppressed, my body was plagued with chronic inflammation that wouldn't quit, I still had more body fat than I wanted, I wasn't getting stronger, and I was only in my late 20s. Worse, I took if for granted that I was condemned to this condition, that my body was the best it could be, given my genes, and that maintaining this level of "fitness" was only going to get harder as I got older.

I was very, very wrong. I was misinformed, and before you shed another ounce of sweat, I think it's worth it for you to stop and consider whether you are misinformed, too. I want to share with you—if only just as food for thought—my take on health, weight loss, and exercise, and some of the "common knowledge" misinformation bombs that are being bandied about in the world of fitness.

Misinformation Bomb #1: The only way to lose fat is to cut calories/burn more calories than you consume.

Even if the calorie is a scientifically worthwhile measure of a food's value, practically it is so one-dimensional as to make it not only almost useless, but also dangerously misleading. I usually describe the problem by saying that the calorie was invented so that Mars Candy could make the argument that a Snickers bar is equivalent, food-value-wise, to a calorically-equal portion of steak. Obviously we know this isn't the case, and yet the calorie-in/calorie-out version of things says it is. So what is Self-Motivated Sam to think?

The calorie-in/calorie-out model isn't entirely inaccurate, but it is woefully incomplete. It ignores the kind of chronic over-storage many Americans create by subsisting on simple carbohydrates in an insulin loop (Sammy Snickers Bar eats something packed with simple carbohydrates, his blood sugar spikes, his body pumps out some insulin, and that sugar gets ferreted away as fat). Worse, it ignores the kind of damage that these simple-sugar foods do to my body. On a technical level, can I eat a Snickers bar and then go run it off? Yes and no: I can "run off" the calories, but I cannot "run off" the cascade of metabolic repercussions. Thus we mistake ill people with artificially suppressed body fat (elevated body fat is only one symptom of an unhealthy diet, folks!) for paragons of "health."

On a personal level, I cringe whenever I see or hear an ad extolling the virtues of a product "with zero calories!" On a very basic level, the calorie is a measure of the energy that can be gleaned from a food: we have become so detached from this definition that we are willing to 1) work (burn calories) to 2) earn money, which we 3) spend on food that is more expensive because it has fewer calories— less energy—and invariably fewer nutrients, etc.

Anybody else see a problem? Am I taking crazy pills?

If you love the idea of calories in/calories out, or it's so ingrained in your thinking that you can't hope to exorcise it, then see if you can at least start thinking of it in terms of carbs in/carbs out. And don't eat Snickers bars.

Misinformation Bomb #2: Long-phase cardio (i.e. running StairMaster/Elliptical) is the best way to lose fat.

False. Completely. Numerous studies have shown that long-phase cardio promotes fat storage by eliciting a cortisol response. So the more you run, the harder it's going to be to lose that weight.

I used to get into arguments with runner friends of mine about this. Again, at the end of the day, doing pretty much anything is better than doing nothing, and if you enjoy running then by all means, run. Just don't go into it expecting something that isn't coming. Similarly:

Misinformation Bomb #3: Running is the best way to build cardiovascular capacity/endurance.

Yes, running is a great way to build cardiovascular endurance... for running. If you run marathons or play soccer, then running makes sense as a training tool. If you participate in combat sports, running is worse than useless: It actually takes time and energy away from other useful forms of training.

Again, it's a question of usage and intention. And, to some extent, it's a question of baseline fitness. General cardiovascular stress (like that achieved by running) can be useful to condition the heart muscle to the increased demands of any activity. However, once a baseline threshold is achieved, running can (and should) be eschewed for more productive forms of training that more closely replicate the demands of the chosen sport.

The kind of intermittent-intensity, multi-movement-pattern stress that you experience in an MMA bout or a Jiu-Jitsu match is a far cry from the constant, single-movement stress of running.

Misinformation Bomb #4: Cardio training is separate from weight training/Cardio means being able to work when you're out of breath/Cardio means conditioning yourself to need less oxygen.

When I look back at my years of training, it astounds me how much time and energy I put into "training cardio" without ever actually considering what the word meant.

When we talk about "cardio," what we're really talking about is supply and demand. My muscles require oxygen to perform work. My blood is the supply stream, carrying that oxygen to my muscles. My heart is the pump that pushes the oxygenated blood to the muscles and draws the deoxygenated blood back to the supply depot. My lungs are the supply depot. They're where my blood goes to pick up more oxygen.

Most of the "cardio" training I see involves creating a greater and greater demand for oxygen by taxing the muscles harder and faster. Some of it even involves impeding the breathing process to exacerbate the deficit. Accordingly, many of us get good at creating a demand, and leave our bodies to catch up and adapt to provide an adequate supply. We become fantastic demanders, and only adequate suppliers.

Once we get a clear picture of what "cardio" actually means, it becomes very clear that a big piece missing from this puzzle is the breath. Simply put: How good are we at breathing?

I know what you're thinking: "Hey, I've been breathing since I was born, and I must be pretty good at it, because I'm still here!" Right? Not quite.

There is plenty of awesome information about this out there, and I'm not going to get into it here, but the long and the short of it is: the greater portion of the blood that passes through your lungs passes through the lower portions, the portions that upper chest breathing (what we usually achieve when we pant for breath, or breathe through our mouths) doesn't access. Breathing nasally into the diaphragm produces significantly more oxygenation than mouth breathing into the upper lungs.

Basically: breathing is a skill, and it is possible to get good at it, and that is where some of the greatest "cardio" gains can be achieved.

Misinformation Bomb #5: Do this exercise to tone the arms/legs/abs/butt!

Ah, toning exercises, the sea route to Asia of the exercise world. Has anybody ever had success toning anything with a toning exercise?

Muscle tone, or muscle definition, is the result of low body fat, period, end of sentence. Low body fat is a result of a good diet, period, end of sentence. "Toning" happens in your kitchen or it doesn't happen at all. "Toning exercises" abound not because they work, but because health and fitness magazines need new content every month.

Misinformation Bomb #6: Scott, you only look the way you do because you train all the time.

I train Jiu-Jitsu almost every day, yes, but it's important for anyone trying to get a sense of what I do to understand the nature of that training. These days for me, rolling is very light and relaxed. I rarely get myself out of breath, and my heart rate rarely gets significantly elevated. Maybe there's a heated exchange here or there, but overall the hour I spend on the mats is easy, more like playing.

I do two strength and conditioning sessions a week. These are usually high-intensity interval training circuits, and usually run no longer than 45 minutes.

I'm 31 years old. I was always a little chunky as a kid. I look the way I look because of how I eat. If you come to class and you workout with me on Monday and Wednesday, you are doing the same amount of hard training I am doing. If you don't like what you see when you take a long, hard look in the mirror, then it's time to take a long, hard look at what's in your refrigerator.

There are more, but this post is running a little long. I'll outline some more of my favorites in the coming weeks. For now, I'll wrap up by saying that if you are one of the Self-Motivated Sams out there, I salute you. I wrote this post for you. If you're finding yourself stuck in a rut, not making any progress or even losing ground, I encourage you to scrutinize the platform on which your routine is founded. Where did that information come from, and is it playing out in your experience? Is it giving you what you want? Is it doing what it promised? If it isn't, don't be afraid to make a radical change.

Stay super.

STOP WORKING OUT, START WORKING IN

Originally published on SuperheroSimplified.blogspot.com
October 21, 2013

The Elephant Story

I had an English teacher in high school who liked to describe how, when it's young, a circus elephant is chained to an immovable post. He explained how, as the elephant grows, a rope is substituted for the chain, and a stake pounded into the ground is substituted for the post. Soon the elephant's restraints seem laughably inadequate: it would take almost no effort at all for the massive elephant to break free. The elephant, however, never breaks free. It learned at a young age that it wasn't strong enough to break its tether (then the chain and post), and after a certain point gave up and stopped trying.

He liked to use this metaphor to describe us, his students. He felt we were too docile, too willing to accept the often absurd corralling imposed on us by parents and school administrators, too willing to allow these restraints to integrate themselves into our perception of ourselves, too willing to enforce the rule of the restraint preemptively, against ourselves.

"I can't do _____," we would think, and soon it became unclear whether this inability arose from some external imposition or if it was rather a quality inherent to ourselves.

41

Thinking About Thinking About Yourself

Nick Carraway, in Fitzgerald's The Great Gatsby, offered the definition of personality as "an unbroken series of successful gestures." In that same vein I like to think of personality as an unbroken series of congruous thoughts about ourselves. Jerry the Jokester thinks of himself as a funny guy, and places emphasis on those moments (in memory and in his day-to-day life) that affirm this self-image. Stuart the Smartypants remembers most those moments when his superior intelligence made the difference.

Jerry and Stuart and all of us imagine ourselves as we wish to appear, work to manifest that image, and then bolster that image with moments of successful implementation: moments in which we successfully appear as we wish to seem.

Conversely, we may be told what we are. "You can't ride your bike to the corner store," we're told by a parent, and (if we're of a certain disposition) this denial may ferment and come to define us to ourselves: the effort and danger of this mission are greater than us, we are insufficient for the imagined task. Each new obstacle presents another opportunity for us to enact the script of our self, to manifest the inferiority we see as the definitive characteristic of our innate, true self.

The manifestations of these self-definitions are so woven into the fabric of our lives, our relationships, our day-to-day interactions that we don't think to notice them. Nor do we consider the manufactured nature of the self: rather, we imagine that this collection of conditioned responses, of situation-specific gestures—this image we continuously create and continuously reenforce—is a set point, a fixed quantity, an unchanging "I" which receives experience and dispenses reactions in accordance with its internal, hard-wired, nature. If we reflect at all, it is often only to conclude with a shrug (or a shout) that, "This is just who I am."

Of course, this is a luxury afforded to those of stable means in stable circumstances. The mental apparatus with which we seek out external reference points and define ourselves in relation to those points in normal life ("I hate going to the mall," "I don't like Nickelback," etc.) is the same apparatus that allows us to normalize during extreme experiences. We are social creatures: despite our mothers' best efforts ("If your friends jumped off a bridge, would you?") we tend to become what we're surrounded by. No matter what we would like to believe, normal people just like us do commit war crimes; law-abiding churchgoers do participate in riots; good kids do, in fact, do dumb, sometimes illegal, things. Our impulse to demonize the guilty, to mentally exile them and amputate them from the body of we, us, the good people, is a mistake, and a terrible waste, because it is exactly their sameness, their similarity to us, that can teach us the most about ourselves, and what it is to be human.

Despite the sometimes horrifying particulars, what these cases suggest to us is that the self is not a fixed quantity. The unbroken series of congruous thoughts that we hold sacred and call ourselves is allowed to persist only in the calm of calamity's indifference, in the safe confines of our staid and regimented and familiar lives. Given some extreme circumstance, would we do the same? And if we did, how would we account for it? Would we assert, as we often hear from the accused, "I don't know what came over me," or, "Things got out of hand," or, "That wasn't me, I'm a good person"? Would we see our misdeed as an aberration, an isolated and singular incongruous act forcing an isolated and singular incongruous thought? Would we attempt to convince ourselves that this incongruous thought does not undermine our years and years of effort, building the house of cards we call ourselves?

Stop Working Out, Start Working In

All of that is a much bigger subject than I have any intention of going into here (and anyway I can't really do it justice: read Malcolm Gladwell's *Blink* if you want more). This post is more concerned with self-ascribed and self-enforced limitation, and how it's a waste of your time and life energy.

As I've said in a previous post, one of the core concepts of my ethic (in the gym and in my life) is that growth and progress only come through failure, that it is only by forcing ourselves past the limits of our current capacity that we are forced to adapt. This is true of exercise, of learning, of anything. We have to face what we do not know or cannot do if we hope to one day know it or do it. The difficulty that arises is that most of us are taught from a very young age that failure—in sports, academics, etc.—is something negative: we laud winners and mock losers; we punish bad grades and reward good grades in an attempt to incentivize success. But in these early, formative trials it is overly easy for events to become definitions: a bad first outing on the field or a bad test score soon convinces us that we're innately "not good at sports," or "not good at math," or "lazy," or physically or mentally "slow." We carry these definitions around with us for years, convincing ourselves with each new failure in the same venue of that definition's intrinsic truth ("See?" we tell ourselves and others. "I told you I was no good at _____.") Slowly we shy away from those venues in which we fail, and those skills and activities that hold the most potential for growth remain untried.

I deal with a lot of people in my role as a coach and a trainer, and I see failure all the time, and too often I see this failure come to negatively dominate the student's experience. "I'm not a natural athlete," I hear them say. Or, "I just don't get it." Or, "I'm not very flexible." Or, "I'm not naturally very strong." I watch their eyes glaze over, and watch as these failures become just more items to add to the list of inferiorities they carry around in their heads. And then I see these people not come back.

Listen. You are only what your previous challenges have forced you to become. There is nothing permanent about any of it. If an infant possessed the mental faculties to compose a self-image, would his or her negative self-judgement ("I'm not a very good walker/talker,") cause him or her to become less likely to try? And would he or she then lag behind developmentally? Of course this example is absurd, but it is no less absurd than what millions of people do to themselves every day, telling themselves that they "are" one way or another, and avoiding doing exactly those things which would make them something else.

If you are one of the many, many people who feel that wave of intimidation and aversion when you think about coming to the gym —feel the fear that you won't be able to do something and that this will be somehow unforgivable, or too shameful to bear—then let me reassure you. In my gym, the only unforgivable sin is wasting time, and the only way to waste time is to put in a day that doesn't encourage you to grow—basically, to put in a day without failure.

You will adapt to the challenges that you present to yourself. The only way for you to be a fixed sum, a changeless point of failure, is to stop trying.

Or, let me say it to you this way: You are the elephant, and your self-assessment is the rope. If you don't test this perceived limit, then it is the strongest restraint that was ever created. But if you test it, I think you will find that it is not so strong after all.

Let go of your emotional attachment to the comfort of "knowing" your own limit. You have to be willing to believe, if only in the context of doing one more stupid push-up, in the power of your own innate potential, your own incredible capacity for change.

You are not a fixed sum. Become super.

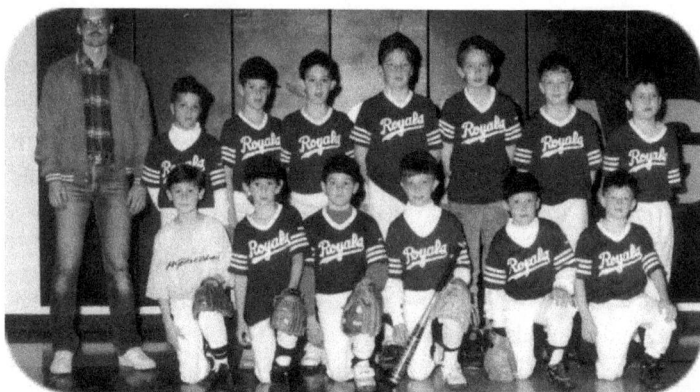

I DON'T BELIEVE IN TALENT

Originally published on SuperheroSimplified.blogspot.com
October 28, 2013

That's me in the front row, the only kid in a colored undershirt. I'm hating every minute of this, because—despite my perpetual hope that, like Superman, I will suddenly develop some unexplainable, freakish athletic ability—I am still terrible at sports.

Early on in my childhood, I can remember parents and teachers telling me and my peers what our own and each others' talents were. "He's such a talented artist," they said about one child. "He's got a lot of musical talent," they said about another. And, "He's a natural athlete," and, "He's a born performer."

These observations turned into decisions. The gifted athletes were encouraged to try out for sports, while the gifted artists were given colored pencils and paint sets for birthdays and Christmases. The parents of the talented musician bought a piano, while the performer's parents signed him or her up for summer drama camp. "Would you like to try _____?" the parents asked, prodding the gifted children in the direction of their gifts. "I think you might really enjoy _____."

Maybe you had a similar experience. I imagine you did. Growing up in middle America, this process was (and I suspect remains) a major part of every child's early integration into larger social settings. The artistic kids gathered in art classes and developed their own micro-society, while the athletic kids played sports together and the drama kids did plays, et cetera.

This corralling is done, I'm sure, with the best of intentions. Parents simply want to see their children thrive, want to see them succeed, want to see them develop confidence in themselves and their abilities. Certainly there are cases where the parental push goes too far, where it exceeds the child's interest, where the parent becomes addicted to the praise heaped on the child, but I'm sure that these aberrations are just that (our current obsession with pageant mothers notwithstanding), and I am less concerned with these dark inversions than I am with the more benignly negative impacts of this seemingly innate part of middle-American child-hood.

As I touched on in last week's post (*Stop Working Out, Start Working In*), these early definitions very fluidly transform from parental assertions (a child's parent perceives a musical/athletic/academic/artistic talent) to societal definition (the parent's friends and the child's peers are presented with the definition of the child, and given opportunities to see him or her in that context) to self-definition (early successes, combined with the general social acceptance of the child's musical/artistic/theatrical talent, informs the child's perception of himself or herself).

The problem arises when one considers that these definitions, no matter how lovingly rendered or asserted, easily imply a limit. The concept of talent carries the implication that, just as an individual has innate abilities, he or she also has innate shortcomings. "I'm good at sports," the child may decide, after encountering less success in the academic realm, "but I'm just not good at math." Or, "I'm a good reader, but I'm not very good at art."

My issue here is not the suggestion that people have shortcomings (people obviously have shortcomings), but rather the sense of the accordant intractability of those shortcomings. One grows up with the sense that he is good at drawing, that artistic talent is an innate component of his makeup, but that (since his proclivities are set) his or her difficulties with sports are equally inescapable.

Talent isn't an intrinsically valuable phenomenon: it doesn't appear on the field or the stage and manifest success. It manifests itself through the artful application of specific skills—skills which are learned, not inborn. But too often it seems that this simple fact is lost behind our resignation to the self as an inescapable fixed quantity: Child X thinks of himself or herself as being inherently bad at sports, and so ignores the fact that the vast majority of his or her supposedly innate incompetence is really just his or her ignorance of specific, learnable skills. Whichever of these skills fall within the scope of Child X's potential (I suspect all) too often remain unexplored: Child X has already resigned himself or herself to his or her present level of ability, and the negative self-definition is proven not by its truth, but rather by Child X's willful subjugation to it.

People I meet nowadays are often surprised to hear that I wasn't an athletic child, that I hated team sports and felt I had no natural aptitude for sport-specific skills. "What sports did you play in high school?" they ask me, assuming I played more than one. Or, after I finish teaching a class on takedowns: "Where did you wrestle?" They seem thrown by my reply that I didn't play any sports, that I started martial arts when I was seventeen, and that I didn't learn to wrestle until I was in my mid-twenties.

I run into people my own age, and I am often astounded by the lives they've created for themselves. Child X grew up, pursued his or her various talent, and eventually went away to college to achieve some higher level of socially-recognized competence in his or her chosen field. He or she was lucky and got a job related to his or her skill set, and this afforded him or her the luxury of economic stability. So he or she purchased a home, and filled his or her off hours with various entertainments, distractions, and hobbies, and at thirty years old Child X has already become the person he or she will be, barring accident or illness, for the next forty to fifty years.

Child X may be happy and healthy and fulfilled. He or she may have built his or her life to his or her exact specifications. But too often I fear the opposite is true: that Child X's life is the product not of willful, intentional construction but rather submission, acceptance, and resignation: the sense that, "I am what I am, this is my place in the world." Peers, advertising, coworkers, bosses, all assert or reinforce in a thousand subtle ways Child X's position, and Child X is soon wholly convinced that his or her current position in the strata of existence is a set, immovable enclosure.

This is not a post about following your dreams, about shaking yourself free of a repressive society. This post is to remind you that you have as much right as anyone else to be good at anything. You are not innately disallowed from any aspect of human endeavor. There is no entrance exam you have to pass.

This is my coaching philosophy. In terms of athletic endeavor (and life in general) talent—innate ability, nature, constitution, whatever you want to call it—is a worthless concept. If talent exists and if you've got it, it's not going to be enough (ask any successful talented person how much of their success can be attributed to their talent, and they'll tell you that talent is nothing without hard work, discipline, and luck). If it exists and you don't have it, then it still doesn't help you one iota to decide that your potential is limited—and to decide even on the specific limits of that potential—before you even start trying. All it does is warm your mind up to the idea of quitting. Locate the concept of talent in your own thinking, in your own sense of yourself and others, take the good and the bad things that branch from it, and chuck it all out of your brain.

Instead, focus with no expectation—either good or bad—on only what you can do today. If you can suspend your habitual sense of your own limitations, I think your true potential just might surprise you.

Get super.

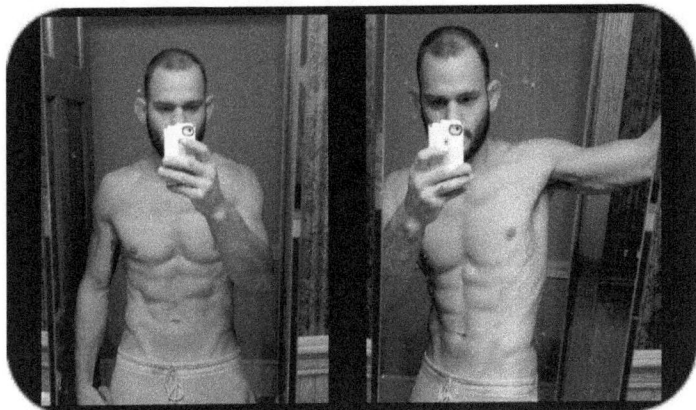

SUPERHERO ABS

Originally published on SuperheroSimplified.blogspot.com
November 3, 2013

NOTE: Yeah. I know. Bathroom mirror selfies are totally obnoxious.

Skills are nice, and self-improvement can be rewarding, but I know that some of you are only here for some inside info on how to look good in your skivvies. Luckily for you, this week's post shows you the ONLY exercise you need to sculpt superhero-caliber abs.

Go to any magazine rack anywhere in the country, and you'll find fitness magazines chock-full of abdominal exercises. This exercise will help you get ripped, washboard abs, one magazine promises. You'll shed unsightly belly fat and develop a slim waistline and sexy, toned core, another claims. We buy these magazines drunk on the belief that we've found the missing piece of the puzzle, that the body we want is one easy, simple modification away. We go into the gym full of gusto, armed with our new guaranteed information, feeling like our goal is well within reach. Soon, a day's work turns into a week's effort, then a month's, and whatever progress we observed in the beginning grinds to a frustrating halt. Are we doing something wrong? Where's the sleek, rippling six-pack we were promised? Luckily, next month's issue has a new batch of ab-torching exercises sure to shake us out of that rut and boost our progress into overdrive...

And so we beat on, boats against the current, borne ceaselessly back into doughy purgatory.

If you came here for the tricks and tips Super Scott uses to get superhero abs, and you thought I was going to show you a variation on the sit-up, think again. What you're going to get in this post is the one piece of insider information you need to know about muscle definition. And that is: There is no such thing as a "toning" exercise.

Imagine a house with a beautifully landscaped front yard. There are tiered beds edged in with river stones and there are rare plants and there are paths and walkways and whatever you think makes a nice yard. All of the edges are clean and all of the elements work together. Then, since this is Cleveland, imagine it's mid-December, with eight inches of lake-effect snow over everything. How well can you see any of that beautiful landscaping?

Yeah. Not very clearly. Exactly.

But you put in all that time and effort, and you want to see your landscaping! So you have a couple options. You can keep constant vigil, and melt whatever snow falls all winter long, you can wait for the environmental conditions to change so that the snow goes away, or you can make all of the elements bigger.

Wait, that third one doesn't make much sense, does it? I mean, even if the stone walls are two feet high instead of a foot high, won't they still be hard to see? Won't they still be covered with the same eight inches of snow?

Yes. Yes they will. And this is the same problem with your doughy gut. Because the fact of the matter is, you have a six pack right now. Everybody does. Yours is probably just buried under a layer of snow.

But Super Scott—I hear you say—isn't that why I'm exercising? I'm going to build a fire in my body and melt away all of that snow! If I combine approaches one and three, I'll have a clear yard in no time.

Yeah, but... Here's the thing. It's *winter*. And it's *Cleveland*. And if you want to keep your landscaping clear, you're going to have to keep that fire going a lot. Like, all winter long. The snow is going to keep falling, and you're going to keep running outside at two in the morning to stoke the embers. I'm not saying that won't give you the yard you always wanted, but I am saying that you won't have time in your life to do much else. And you will be exhausted.

Or you can move south. And by "move south," I mean stop putting the stuff in your mouth that makes the "snow" fall and collect on your "yard."

Winter is an environmental condition like your diet is an environmental condition.

Have I beaten this metaphor to death yet?

The dirty little secret of the "fitness" (read: exercise) industry is that diet has way, way more to do with body composition than ANYTHING you do in the gym. Yes, diet and exercise are the essential ingredients of any weight-loss plan, but saying it like that ("diet and exercise") sometimes seems to imply that the two are of equal importance and this, I think, allows many of us to believe that, since each makes up half of the whole picture, more investment in exercise can make up for less investment in diet. Take it from me: It doesn't work like that. Yes, the formula for weight loss is diet and exercise, but the full version of that formula is more like nine parts diet to one part exercise. You need to fix your diet if you want to see your abs. End of story.

Take a look at the picture at the top of this post. I took that picture on Wednesday of last week. I worked out Monday, and as part of my workout I did 120 seated twists (sitting with my legs held off the ground and twisting side to side, shoulders and legs going opposite directions) and I held the boat pose for a total of one minute and 15 seconds. Those were the only core-specific exercises I did. My last workout before that was on the previous Wednesday, where my only core-specific exercise was 63 v-ups, broken up into 21-rep sets.

Those are the ONLY core-specific exercises I did in those seven days, and those numbers are very typical for me.

During that same time period I ate only plants (fruits and vegetables), meats, and cultured dairy (cheese and yogurt). I ate when I was hungry, and I ate until I was full, and I even (since my Sidekick didn't get home from work until after ten on some nights) ate late at night.

As important as what I did eat, though, is what I didn't eat. I ate no refined sugar or processed carbohydrates. I ate nothing from the center of the grocery store.

So what's the one and only exercise I promised you at the beginning of this post? It's diagramed in detail on the next page. When you find yourself reaching for the refined sugar and junk carbs, "exercise" some self-control and eat something else. That's the smart, easy, sustainable, and truly healthful way to alleviate the environmental conditions that cause the "snow" to keep collecting on your "yard."

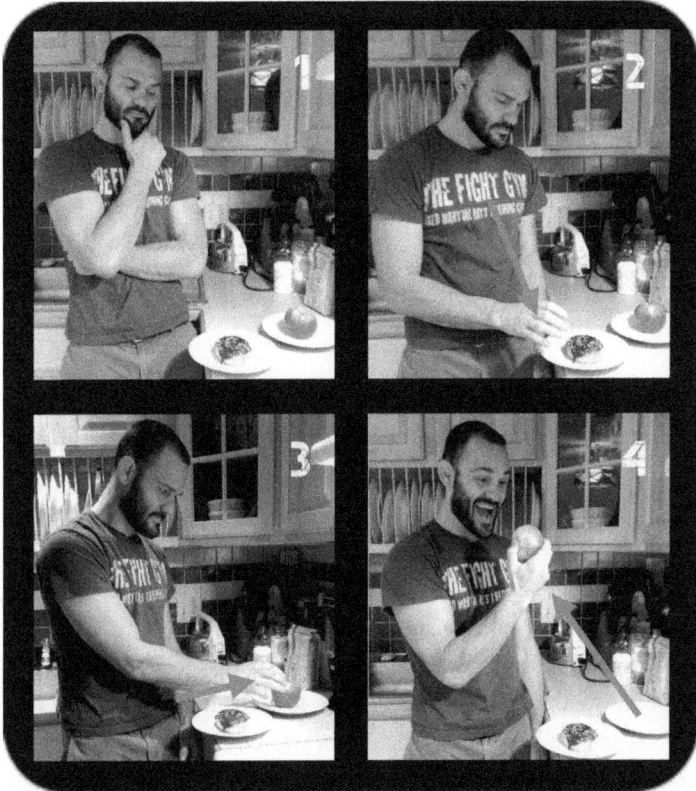

1. Our hero is facing a crisis! What to eat to satisfy his super hunger?
2. Our hero reaches for the donut...
3. ...but with a burst of superhuman effort, he narrowly escapes disaster!
4. Our hero emerges victorious once again.

Stay super.

PUT DOWN THAT CUPCAKE, CUPCAKE

Originally published on SuperheroSimplified.blogspot.com
November 11, 2013

For many of us, food carries heavy emotional weight. Some of these associations are intrinsic—warm food is comforting on a cold day; sweet food is pleasurable to eat—but often the associations are far more subtle, and far more difficult to recognize and unpack. Perhaps when we were young ice cream was our parents' reward for a good grade on a test. Maybe when we were bad and fought with our siblings, we were sent to bed without dessert.

Food is an essential need and, as with any essential need, the emotions associated with it run deep and strong, and often run entirely beneath the level of any intervention from our conscious mind. Consider: a common childhood experience is that of being held accidentally (or intentionally) underwater while swimming: perhaps you remember your body's frantic, animal response to the denial—or perceived threat of denial—of life-giving oxygen. How closely did you later examine that experience, or critique your own response? Chances are that you didn't consider it very much, that you feel your response was justified, no matter what it was, and that the aversion you feel toward the memory of the experience and your own unpleasant panic and fear have subtly encouraged you not to reconsider it.

This fear/panic response is a key ingredient in our ongoing survival as individuals and as a species, but it is not overly attuned to its circumstances. Were you actually drowning when you began to frantically fight? Perhaps you were and perhaps you weren't: the point is that the fear you felt has no degrees: your mind sensed the threat, and triggered the panic procedure with little regard to whether the dunking was friendly horsing around or malevolent attack.

Our modern lives are blessedly free from many of the survival concerns that defined our species for much of its existence. This, however, seems to have hardly dampened the power of our survival/panic response: the so-called "fight or flight" response is always just a speeding car or a misstep on a steep staircase, or even a threatening word, away. We tend to think of this response as arising at moments of impending physical danger, but I think this mechanism defines much more of our lives, and crops up to handle more of our experiences, than we might think.

Imagine, for a second, that you are at a birthday party for a co-worker. You like the co-worker, and you would like to be better friends with her, and you want her friends to like you, but at this point you don't know her friends at all. They've been pleasant enough, but largely seem uninterested in you. The birthday treat comes out. It's cupcakes, and there aren't enough to go around. In fact, there's one more person than there are cupcakes. There should have been enough, but one of the co-worker's friends brought another friend. The cupcakes get handed around, and you watch as one by one everyone bites into theirs without noticing that you didn't get one...

Or imagine that you come to The Fight Gym, and you ask me to help you lose weight, and the first thing I tell you is that you can't eat one certain food, a food which just so happens to be your favorite food. I insist, and I promise you that you can't lose weight without giving up this food.

How do these experiences make you feel? Certainly it is natural to feel excluded, slighted, hurt, forgotten, by the group of friends all eating their cupcakes. Certainly it is easy to feel personally criticized when I say that your favorite food is a no-no. But what is this small, needling panic that crops up as you watch the cupcakes disappear one by one, as you realize that the numbers don't match, as you see the friend's friend reaching to take one? What is this subtle, panicky sense of denial, as you imagine a future bereft of your very favorite food?

Food is just food, and yet for so many reasons, food is so much more. It's a way we give and receive love (anyone's mother cook them their favorite meal as a way of showing her love? Anyone cook a special meal for their child as a way of showing their love?). It's how we commune with one another (and, for some of us, with a higher power). It is a way of literally giving someone a part of yourself (that food was going to become part of you, and instead it's going to become part of whoever you gave it to). It's a way for us to express our creativity, to express our individuality ("I used my special secret recipe," "I used my Grandmother's marinade," etc.).

For these reasons, it is easy to see our food as part of ourselves, as literally an extension of our ego, and I would argue that the threat of denial of specific emotionally weighty foods can feel as viscerally frightening as the threat of the denial of air. We retreat into panicked thinking, withdraw from the source of the denial or maybe even actively attack it (in thought, at least). But of course panicked thinking isn't rational thinking: we aren't going to starve when we get to the break room and see the donut box standing empty any more than we're going to drown when our best friend dunks us under water. It just isn't going to happen.

If you're trying to lose weight and it isn't working, the reason doesn't live in the gym. It lives in your cupboards and in your fridge, or it lives in the break room, or it lives in the Starbucks display case and syrup pumps. It lives in those "little treats" you give yourself because you "had a hard day" or because you've "been so good on your diet lately." If you are serious about losing weight then you need to change your diet, and that means confronting that little irrational voice in your head that starts screaming and crying and throwing its little tantrum when you put the ice cream back in the freezer.

Take my word for it: You're going to be OK without that cupcake. You're going to be ok never eating birthday cake ever again. It's still summer even if you don't have an ice cream cone. Your mother still loves you, even if you don't eat her lasagna. It's still Thanksgiving without pumpkin pie, and it's still Christmas without cookies. It's time to stop being a little kid and losing your mind because someone is offering you or denying you a treat. I don't care that you can only get a Shamrock shake for a few weeks every year. Those weeks can come and go and you'll still be here, even if you don't fill your gut with green-colored goop. I promise you, it's all going to be all right.

Stay super.

CASTAWAY FITNESS

Originally published on SuperheroSimplified.blogspot.com
November 25, 2013

It's 6:20AM here on Kauai. The feral roosters are crowing, and I am wide awake. But it's not the roosters that have me pacing the floor of our little bungalow, nor is it the time change. I'm up and at 'em early this morning because I know I've been falling behind on the blog, and I need to post something for all you aspiring super-heroes out there: something to let you know that even though I'm off the mainland, I have not abandoned you!

As many of you know, I'm here with Steve Maxwell, my Gracie Jiu-Jitsu coach and a widely sought-out authority on health, fitness, mobility, and strength & conditioning (I'm not going to list Steve's resume here, but if you don't know who he is, do a quick YouTube search). We're here filming a series of instructional videos about how to use found objects and natural implements to achieve a killer workout, even when you're far from your home gym and your usual routine.

Hanging out with Steve, as usual, has got me thinking. The sun sets early here, and this gives us plenty of downtime to hang out and chat about Jiu-Jitsu, training, and the current state of American health and fitness. It also gives me the opportunity to sound some of my ideas against Steve's fifty-plus years of training experience, and see where I'm headed in the right direction, and where I'm turned around.

You don't need me to tell you that the current state of our health is a pretty sorry one. Obesity and obesity-related illnesses are rampant, even among the young. There are plenty of theories as to why this has come about: some say it's our increasingly refined-carb-based diet (I would tend to agree); some say it's our increasingly digital, vicarious, avatar-based leisure activities (I can't imagine this is helping the situation); others say it's our culture's general attitude of entitlement, consumption, and permissiveness (don't get me started). However, for the sake of this post, I'm going to give everyone the benefit of the doubt and assume that, for everyone out there who truly doesn't want to work out, there is someone else who wants to work out, but literally doesn't know how.

Those of us who teach skills sometimes have a hard time bridging the gap between what we know and what our pupils don't know, because we literally can't remember what it's like to not know something we've known for so long. I've had teachers who were brilliant at shaping out the space for new information in my brain—prompting me to understand the limit of my abilities first and then showing me how a new technique or procedure will help me achieve the end I couldn't previously manage—and I've had other teachers who simply fed me information without giving me any context in which to house it (guess which one worked better). In this case, in this blog post, I'm going to assume that the issue with the average "unfit American" is not his or her inherent laziness, but his or her entirely forgivable ignorance: namely the fact that despite the myriad resources available, despite the volumes and volumes of fitness magazines and celebrity diet books and equipment fads and gym facilities, no one really ever bothers to tell the Average Joe what "fitness" means, i.e. no one tells him how his body works, and what he needs to do to optimize those abilities.

Think about it. At some point in your life you probably became aware that there were athletes and non-athletes in your elementary school class. There were those who were "physically gifted." You probably remember these athletes running laps around the track, running on the tread mill, lifting in the gym, and training in their sport. You understood that these people were "fit" and you deduced that these methods—these various exercises that you saw them do-ing—were the path to their fitness. Maybe you were one of these athletes yourself, or maybe you worked out with them, and you gleaned from their training a sense of what your own training should be: the "requirements" of physical fitness.

This was my first experience of training. I understood that there was a gap between myself and the athletes without understanding the nature of that gap. I learned their methods, and assumed that these methods would allow me to bridge the gap. But this is a bit like fixing a leaking pipe without knowing quite where the leak is: you can keep applying sealant in the vicinity of the water trickling out, hoping that you'll get lucky and land on the source of the problem. And maybe you do get lucky and the leak stops, and maybe you don't, but either way you don't really know anything about the leak, and you've wasted a lot of time and effort and ma-terial in the trying.

So I'm going to assume that, rather than laziness, it is this igno-rance that causes many the aversion they feel when they think about working out. They look through the gym window and they see the piles and piles of weights and medicine balls and other fitness equipment. They see the specialized machines. They watch celebrity fitness shows and they see various implements employed in various ways for largely unexplained purposes. They understand that these practices are what make people "fit," and they understand that they should be "fit," but they have no one to explain how this mountain of equipment works, nor the time to take on the monumental task of orienting themselves in this world they know little about.

And this, I think, is where many of us trainers fail our clients. We say, "It's easy to work out for thirty minutes a day! If you don't do it, you're lazy!" But of course the task in front of these people is not simply to carve out thirty minutes a day: it is to go back to school, to become a student of exercise equipment and procedure, and it is not hard to imagine that—for many—simply "working out" quickly seems a massive undertaking, an insurmountable obstacle. It really is no wonder, then, that people throw up their hands and stick with what they already understand and are comfortable doing (i.e. eating pizza and playing Xbox).

So I'm going to break it down and give you the simplified owner's manual for the human body, the manual I wish I had when I started working out. Here it is.

Your body is a machine. Muscular elements pull structural elements. The structural elements hinge at joints. The orientation of these muscular elements and these joints determines the range of motion in which any given structural element is designed to move, i.e. your biceps pull your hand toward your shoulder, and your elbow joint determines the track it follows. Your triceps do the opposite.

Every muscle group in your body is designed to help you accomplish (basically) one of seven movements. When you exercise one of these seven movement patterns you engage the whole chain of muscles designed to accomplish that movement, and you can develop strength in each while also developing the collective efficacy of the total movement. These movements are:

1. Overhead push
2. Overhead pull
3. Lateral press
4. Lateral pull
5. Extension with the front thighs
6. Extension with the back, hips, and hamstrings
7. Stabilization (anti-rotation) of the spine

That's your whole body. If you do something to work each of these movements, you will hit every muscle group as well as develop collective strength across the entire range of each motion.

So, how do we work these movements effectively? Here are a few simple suggestions:

1. Overhead push: Do a push-up from downward facing dog, turning your elbows toward the floor and touching your nose in between your hands. Make sure the motion is forward and backward, not just up and down.

2. Overhead pull: Pull-up. Make sure the arms rotate and the elbows point forward—not to your sides—as you pull yourself up to the bar.

3. Lateral press: The humble push-up.

4. Lateral pull: Row. Grip and clamber under something that's about solar plexus height, keep your body stiff like a board, and pull your chest to the bar.

5. Extension with the front thighs: Squat. A body weight squat at high reps can be a fantastic workout in and of itself, but you can easily add "weight" by exploding off the feet at the top of the squat. The added force you generate is comparable to adding an external weight.

6. Extension with the back, hips, and hamstrings: These are the muscle groups that allow you to stand up from bowing or bending forward at the waist, that engage from the heel through the lower and middle back. For this range it's helpful to have an external weight, but think about it: a big stockpot full of water, a rock, a log, etc., can easily be employed for this purpose. You don't need a gym.

7. Stabilization of the spine: This is the core. If you do the rest of these motions properly, you are already doing it. The core should be engaged throughout. You can add a twisting motion, i.e. a stepping twisting lunge, for added engagement, but it really isn't necessary. Remember what I've said in previous posts: six-pack abs aren't made in the gym, they're made in the kitchen.

Now I know what you're thinking: But Scott, what about cardio? Don't I need to run on the treadmill? Don't I need my exer-bike? Don't I need my StairMaster?

Again with the vague attributes! Athletes have great cardio; I want great cardio; I need to do what the athletes do, right? Well, yes and no. First off, take a second to think about what it means to have great cardio. If you're anything like I was for most of my fitness-oriented life, "cardio" meant being able to go harder and faster without getting out of breath, or being able to work harder when I was out of breath, or being able to catch my breath more quickly. The actual mechanics, the actual problem, was largely obscured to me: I understood that I got out of breath when I worked hard, but I didn't understand how it was happening, or what the apparatus was that I was trying to develop.

So let's take it back to basics. Your muscles need oxygen to function. Your blood carries oxygen to your muscles. Your heart pumps the blood from your lungs to your muscles. Your lungs are the supply depot, where oxygen gets picked up and carbon dioxide gets dropped off. Your heart pumps your blood to and from your lungs, to and from your muscles. That's cardio.

So, how do we put greater demand on this system so that my heart muscle gets stronger, the musculature of my respiration gets stronger, the oxygen-carrying capacity of my blood increases, the coordination of the system (and here I'm talking about the actual inhale-exhale practice of breathing) improves? A workout comprised of the seven elements listed above, done at a taxing pace, will give you all the cardiovascular demand you need. Remember, we're talking about the sum total of your functionality as a machine: what more could you need from your cardiovascular system than its efficacy as the supply chain for these inherent human movement patterns?

I hope this gives those of you who are overwhelmed by the prospect of "getting fit" a place to start. And for those of you who already work out—the Self-Motivated Sams out there—I hope this gives you a few ideas you can use. You see that it's not so hard to get all the workout you need with very little equipment.

Until next time, aloha and stay super!

FIGHTING VS. ROLLING

Originally published on SuperheroSimplified.blogspot.com
December 3, 2013

Brazilian Jiu-Jitsu is a combat sport, designed to give people the tools they need to successfully negotiate an altercation. Learning Brazilian Jiu-Jitsu means learning how to fight, and it is because of—and for—this very reason that training (sparring or "rolling") looks so much like fighting.

Fighting keeps a martial art, for lack of a better word, honest. When Royce Gracie stepped into the Octagon in the first Ultimate Fighting Championship twenty years ago, he was stepping in against men whose martial arts were largely limited by the artificial parameters of those styles. In other words, these men trained mostly against opponents whose skill set and strategy mirrored their own: the boxer trained against other boxers, knew how to fight other boxers, knew how to defend boxing attacks and how to manage a boxing-based altercation; he had little to no experience against kicks, or in a grappling situation, or on the ground. His style, though akin to fighting, could not really be called fighting: its limitations made it more closely related to other sporting contests in which athletes compete against each other within a specific set of predetermined parameters.

The Gracies knew that, in a real fight, there are no rules, no sport-specific parameters, and no time limits. Their style of Jiu-Jitsu grew from an organic connection to the variability of real combat, and it is this continuing connection (through MMA and Jiu-Jitsu competition) that keeps Jiu-Jitsu so effective. What works in live practice stays in the art, what doesn't falls by the wayside.

Fighting is an essential part of BJJ training. The ability to success-fully implement techniques against an aggressive and resistant op-ponent is the mark of the skilled practitioner. For practitioners of the art, however, it is a mistake to approach every sparring session as a fight. Even without the use of strikes or other such attacks, a "fight-ing" style of Jiu-Jitsu is rougher and more injurious. Moreover, it can be counterproductive: a novice fighter gains little from a training match in which he is ground into the mat; he learns only that he has much more to learn (a lesson which has its place, certainly, but which also does not need the kind of reteaching which repeated smashing offers).

Inversely, a practitioner who adopts an overly casual or "easy" training demeanor can fail to develop the requisite conditioning and timing a true combat situation may require.

It is for this reason that I encourage practitioners to think of sparring as having two separate characters. "Fighting" is for condi-tioning, for testing oneself and one's skills. It can be a useful training demeanor to have when training with one's peers: those of compa-rable age, size, strength, and ability. A "fight" is not a good environ-ment for experimentation, for attempting new or less familiar tech-niques, because the cost of any mistake is too high. "Fighting" is hard, fast, injurious, and unsustainable: a "fighting" demeanor can-not be maintained for the course of a ten or a fifteen or a twenty minute match without exhaustion. It is akin to the sport of wrestling, in which size, strength, and conditioning are of paramount impor-tance. On the other hand, "rolling" is played like chess. The pace should be somewhat lax and the participants somewhat forgiving.

When "rolling" the rule of thumb is: if you had to change speed or exertion level to make a move work, then you didn't really make it work, because a comparable change in speed or exertion level from your opponent could have arrested it. "Rolling" is fun, more akin to horseplay than a fight, and is the time and place to attempt new moves.

If you train BJJ, I encourage you to approach your sparring sessions with this mentality. Fighting and rolling both offer their own benefits and limitations, and to do either exclusively is a mistake. Let fighting be fighting and rolling be rolling, and decide (with your opponent), on a match-by-match basis, which demeanor to adopt. This of course requires you to find training partners who understand the distinction: when you find them, train with them as much as possible.

If you run a BJJ program, I encourage you to set aside one or two sessions a week for "competition team" training, and several other sessions for open rolling, and explain to your students the appropriate demeanor for each. I firmly believe that this approach will reap the most benefit for everyone, from white to black belt.

EVERYONE IS ENTITLED TO THEIR OPINION, or THE LOST ART OF IGNORANCE

Originally published on SuperheroSimplified.blogspot.com
December 9, 2013

NOTE: I talk about some extreme behaviors in this post, and for this reason it would be easy to dismiss some of what I say. You may find yourself saying, "I never get too bent out of shape when someone takes my parking spot, this blog post isn't talking about me, I don't have any of these tendencies." I encourage you to realize that the extreme behaviors I'm talking about are extreme behaviors, and that what I say here might still be of some relevance to you.

"If a genius does something I don't understand, why do I think he's wrong?"

— Scott Adams

I listen to a lot of programs on NPR, and I am consistently amazed by the number of people who call into talk radio shows to proffer their opinions about a subject to an expert on that subject. Just once I would like to hear the expert reply, "Thank you, Billy-Bob from Nowheresville, Nowhere; your take on the ongoing conflict in the Middle East was the voice that was missing from the discussion. Armed with your insight, I'm certain a sustainable solution is now well within reach."

I'm not the first to say it, but we have a real self-worth problem in this country. Nor am I the first to point out that this may have a lot to do with the fact that we're under nearly constant assault from advertisers, all of them working hard to convince us that our unforgivable and shameful inadequacies can be overcome by the acquisition and ownership of whatever product they're selling. Our economy depends on our ongoing consumption, but for many of us our actual needs have long since been met, so advertisers tickle our (all-too-accessible) fear that we will be left behind, alone, unwanted and unloved.

It's little wonder, then, that we are so violently averse to any interpersonal, ground-level (i.e. person-to-person, as opposed to cultural-level) suggestion that we are inadequate, that we are undeserving of consideration, that we are somehow inferior or fail to meet the minimum standard that would earn us equal regard in the eyes of others. Someone takes our parking spot, or cuts ahead of us in line at the grocery store, or takes the last whatever off the shelf just as we were reaching for it, and we react as though this simple act is an affront to our entire existence. Similarly we may perceive the assertion of another's opinion as an adversarial gesture, may feel at once that our own (contrary) opinion is being overridden by the oppositional declaration, and feel that I, the voice behind the opinion, is being likewise passed over, forgotten, belittled, ignored...

Really, it's no wonder that so many of us express such disproportionate outrage: advertising culture assaults us during nearly every moment of our waking lives, from our computer screens and televisions and car radios and billboards and on and on and on. We live with someone constantly whispering in our ear: "You are not enough as you are." It is little wonder, then, that sooner or later we hunker down within the last defensible position we can imagine: we fortify

71

ourselves within the confines of our "own experience" and reject as illegitimate any ground-level attack: "You can't tell me that I'm not good enough/my opinion is wrong/I don't know enough," we say to any oppositional force we imagine our shouting can overcome. "You don't know what it's like to be me/don't know my story/don't know my genetics/don't know how hard a time I'm having." We seize the meager authority this position offers (after all, no one can claim to be a greater expert on me than me!) and we hold it before us like a shield, obscuring and deflecting anything we find threatening.

Of course this approach is wholly ineffective: the loudness of our cries does not obscure our actual inadequacies. If I don't know how to swim, and someone tries to teach me how to swim, and I instead attack them for their slight (if I perceive that their suggestion—that I need to learn how to swim—is in fact an assertion that I am somehow lacking) and leave before they teach me anything, all the shouting in the world doesn't make up for the fact that I still don't know how to swim.

I've thought a lot about this phenomenon, and I am more and more convinced that it is the result of a cultural belief that, though it was propagated with the best of intentions, has ended up doing far more harm than good. I am talking about the idea that everyone is unique and special, the idea that everyone has different skills and talents, an idea I'm going to refer to as the Snowflake Fallacy.

The Snowflake Fallacy asserts that "you" are a fixed quantity, a set being with attributes, talents, and limitations. Positively, the Snowflake Fallacy asserts that no one else can do exactly what you do, that you are inherently valuable for your own unique allotment of skills, intelligence, etc. Inversely, however, the Snowflake Fallacy carries with it the implication that your limitations are as fixed as your talents, and herein lies the problem, because if I feel that my limitations are inescapable then I can't do anything but defend them when I feel they are being attacked. If I regard my limitations as inherent to myself then I can only feel that myself is being attacked when some limitation is pointed out.

The perception that I am an innately fixed sum is inaccurate. People change all the time, and in drastic and dramatic and fundamental ways. Worse, and more importantly, this perception is wholly unproductive. A limitation defended becomes stuck, guarded, immune to change: does in fact become a permanent attribute *because it is claimed and maintained as one.*

A limitation acknowledged does not grow in proportion to the other aspects of your personhood. Now exposed to outside influence it is subject to the profound altering force of practice, learning, and further experience. The person, the "I" I sought to defend by hiding my inadequacy, was never less than what it always was (for the inadequacy, acknowledged or not, remained the same). Now, the limitation revealed, the "I" can truly grow.

There is no shame in not knowing what you don't know. The shame is in dismissing the unknown in a pathetic attempt to validate a fragile self against a perceived slight. If you meet someone who is an expert on a particular subject, and he or she is willing to take the time to tell you his or her opinion on that subject, it is best to remind yourself that in this particular case you are NOT entitled to your opinion.

JIU-JITSU FOR A BETTER WORLD

Originally published on SuperheroSimplified.blogspot.com
December 30, 2013

If you hang around the Jiu-Jitsu world long enough, you're going to hear people make some pretty hefty claims. I'm not talking about the claims they make about themselves and their abilities, or those of their team or teammates. I'm talking about the claims they make about Jiu-Jitsu and it's power to change the world.

"If everyone did Jiu-Jitsu," they say, "the world would be a better place."

The reasons they give are various. Jiu-Jitsu practitioners have healthier egos, they say, because BJJ practitioners are humbled on a daily basis. Jiu-Jitsu practitioners learn to leave their differences at the door, and learn to treat their best friend and their greatest adversary with the same honor and respect. Jiu-Jitsu practitioners learn to control their emotions and handle stress with intelligence and rationality, which translates into better outcomes in situations at home, in the workplace, on the street, and in all walks of life.

While all of these are valid points, I want to highlight a more basic (and perhaps, somewhat more disquieting) point that often goes unsaid. The inherent truth at the core of Jiu-Jitsu, the one with which practitioners are constantly in contact, is that regardless of your political affiliations, feelings on same-sex marriage, feelings about the Bible as the literal transcription of God's word, favorite reality television programs, least favorite reality television programs, food allergies, relationship with your parents, grades in school, position at your company, adjusted annual gross income, adjusted annual net income, zip code, aspirations, fears, hair color, eye color, weight, gender, race, fashion sense, favorite Beatle, favorite Jonas brother, favorite ninja turtle, favorite brand of caffeinated energy drink, level of education—regardless of all of this, you are a bag of guts whose elbows and knees bend one way and not the other, whose brain needs a steady supply of oxygenated blood, whose muscles tire when they exceed their work capacity, whose soft tissues tear when they get stretched past their limit.

The real basic insight of Jiu-Jitsu is that despite all of our claimed differences we are uniform in our naked human limitation. All too often I see practitioners who view the martial arts as a kind of super power: I know something you don't know, I know how to hurt you and you don't know how to hurt me, and this makes me some kind of superman, unlike everyone else. To me, this view wholly misses the point: BJJ is not about building up your own strength, about making yourself more powerful so that you can have it over on someone else. BJJ is about understanding your own limitations, and through understanding yourself in this way, understanding everyone else in this way, too.

Everyone is weak. Everyone is limited. Everyone is bound by the parameters of the human body. We, as a species, stand on this planet before all of its incredible forces with only these meager, human attributes to defend and bolster and maintain and propagate ourselves.

It is a luxury of modern, and particularly modern American, society that most of us don't have to confront our own weakness on a daily basis: that we somehow feel that we alone are enough to stand in the world. We build separate houses and we live like islands that occasionally contact one another, thinking that if things ever went wrong we could blockade ourselves inside our own private kingdoms and ward off the coming storm with our own strength or fortitude or cunning. This, however, is a ridiculous delusion: the forces in life and in nature operate on a scale that is vast beyond our reckoning, and our small-minded assertions about them (i.e. "The tornado won't hit my house, because a tornado is bad, and I'm good,") compel them not in the least.

People who really get Jiu-Jitsu understand this. They understand that conflict is born of a certain breed of insanity which allows me to ignore the profound horror I should feel when I see another person suffering: an insanity which allows me to believe that this suffering could never befall me, that the sufferer is some other kind of creature unlike myself. People who really understand Jiu-Jitsu understand that we must be merciful to one another because one day we too may stand exposed in our weakness, and we will then depend on the mercy of others. They understand that the human race in sum is not much to stand against the myriad forces that threaten to blot it out.

I do believe that Jiu-Jitsu has the power to make the world better, but only when its practitioners move beyond the pursuit of some personal glory, some vision of individual superhuman power. It can change the world when its participants understand that every weakness they exploit on an opponent is their own: that no asserted superficial difference can mask our innate human sameness. It can change the world when we all understand that Jiu-Jitsu is a meditation on our own weakness, and we let that knowledge compel us toward mercy.

CARE VS. WORRY, OR
HOW I LEARNED TO STOP
WORRYING AND LOVE THE LOVE

Originally published on SuperheroSimplified.blogspot.com
January 27, 2014

"I know they're being foolish. All farmers ever do is worry, whether the rain falls, the sun shines, or the wind blows. In short, all they know is fear. Their behavior today is also due simply to fear."

—The Old Man, Kurosawa's *Seven Samurai*

My name is Scott, and I have something to confess. I'm a worrier.

The funny thing is, until recently, I didn't really realize that I was a worrier. I knew I worried (about the noise my car was making, about the money I just spent, about my health, about a million unlikely hypotheticals), but I always chalked it up to my being "responsible" and "grounded": to the fact that I was an "intelligent person" who "thought ahead."

Maybe you're like me. Maybe you also worry, and maybe you even consider your worry the mark of an underlying virtue: "I worry about my wife/girlfriend/friend/child because I care about them," we tell ourselves. "I worry about my financial future because I'm on the ball, handling my responsibilities."

But what is worry, really? And what are these (sometimes vague, sometimes highly specific) hypothetical situations we dream up to torment ourselves?

One of the big differences between Brazilian Jiu-Jitsu and many other martial arts, I often tell people, is that by incorporating live, free-form sparring into training, BJJ practitioners have the opportunity to train not only their physical techniques, but the unique skill involved in engaging these techniques in a stressful, adrenalized state. BJJ training, if done mindfully, can more closely replicate the internal state (high heart-rate, panic breathing, racing thoughts) of an actual confrontation, and the student must then learn to deal with the physical and mental products of stress. (BJJ is not the only martial art that affords its students this opportunity, but it is among a small number, a startling fact when one considers that this skill—the management of stress—is likely the vital difference between success and failure in an actual confrontation.)

To put it another way, BJJ students learn to deal with fear. They learn fear's true physical detrimental effects: the racing heart-rate, the hyperventilation, the adrenaline rush and subsequent debilitating fatigue, the rapid decline in motor function, the panicked thinking. They learn to deal with fear not by ignoring it or imagining themselves above it, but by understanding it: understanding it as part of the danger of a situation, and working to guard themselves against it just as they guard themselves against the assailant.

I've been doing BJJ for a while now, and I thought I was pretty good at this particular skill. Moreover, it was a point of pride for me: that I understood BJJ to be more than just a physical contest; that real self-defense came in understanding the limits of both your body and your mind; that defending yourself against the detrimental (and often defeat-producing) effects of panic was as central to the art as defending an armlock or a choke.

It didn't occur to me until very recently that—while I could be calm, cool, and vigilant on the mats—fear was getting the better of me in pretty much every other part of my life. My car would make a funny noise, or I would try to plan a trip, and suddenly my mind would be off and running, formulating dozens of potential futures in which events conspired against me: in which any gap in my planning proved disastrous.

As I said, up until recently, I considered this a virtue. I thought it was a mark of my reliability or my intelligence. Now, however, I see it for what it is: the habitual mental process of someone who has let fear run amuck, who fears the future and so attempts to preempt its disasters with premature emotional fortitude, or thinks that—like some ancient tribal ritual used to ward off evil—these thoughts will somehow divert the track of the calamity I fear is headed my direction.

The danger here is not that these mental gyrations will keep me from doing anything I might otherwise do. The danger here is that I don't enjoy things I would otherwise enjoy: that I experience the thing or the event or the person as only a series of stress triggers: my care or love gets immediately diverted into worry. Instead of being suffused with the biology of affection or love or care (that natural high of pleasure chemicals) I am awash in the biology of fear (adrenaline, muscular tension, elevated heart rate, etc.). What's worse, this mental move (allowing care to turn into worry) gets easier and easier the more I practice it, soon making it impossible for me to feel the energizing effect of love without using that energy as fuel for concern.

I'm sharing this because I think you're probably like me, because fear-mongering is America's true national pastime. Recalling the dim specter of "potential calamity" (whether that calamity is a home invasion or social alienation) is the best and oldest way to sell people stuff that they don't (currently) need. You may not need this product now, advertising likes to tell us, but what about in the future? Imagine a future in which you do need it! What if you don't have it then? What a disaster that would be! Care (about what your lawn is going to look like this summer, about making new friends at school, about what your dream girl is going to think of you, about where you're going to retire) gets translated into fear via various and specific potential undesirable outcomes (your lawn looks terrible, you don't make any friends, the girl laughs at you), and we're left scrambling to buy enough duct tape to stave off the anthrax attack.

This entire apparatus of turning care into fear insidiously convinces us that worry is the appropriate activity of care. We're told and become convinced (as I was, as a kid) that worrying is the mark of someone who thinks ahead, who plans, who has his feet on the ground, who has a good head on his shoulders. Maybe we hear it at home as well: "I worry because I care!" our mothers say. Or sometimes, the more unsettling version: "I worry about you," which leaves us to extrapolate the care that prompted the statement, further blurring the lines in our fear-soaked mind between care (positive, pleasurable, healthy) and concern (toxic, stressful, unhealthy).

So the question becomes: Am I ready to stop worrying? Am I ready to let care and love exist as care and love, and nourish me, without subverting them into fear? And if not, why not? What value is worry adding to my life, that I am loathe to relinquish?

The answer, I think, is that worry seems to lay the groundwork for a more successful future. If I think ahead—like the ant in the story, who stores food away for the winter—I will endure more effectively when that calamity does come. Or I will avoid the calamity altogether by identifying potential pitfalls. But to me now, these seem like poor offerings: not because they are not valuable in themselves, but because care is capable of producing these same effects. When you care about something (your health, your kid, your car, your leaky roof) you invest your energy in it. You cultivate its *present* state. And a successful and thriving present is enough because the phenomenal truth is that *the future never comes*. You will always only experience the present.

Or think about it this way: worry is the thief that steals the present moment—that elusive present moment—that all of us are always trying to live in.

Care prepares. Care performs the acts of care. Care is present, and a present that shows the mark of care will show the mark of care tomorrow and the day after and the day after that. Worry, that fear of the future, is a waste of not just time: it is a waste of love.

So don't worry. Be happy. Not because there's nothing to worry about, but because worry is worthless. It doesn't mean that you don't *have* worries, it means that you've chosen not to worry in the same way you would choose not to eat cupcakes, hang out with dangerous people, go into bad neighborhoods. It is an intentional refusal of a negative and potentially destructive practice that, in the end, offers no rewards to justify itself in the first place.

It's a frightening thing, to live in a state of open-ended, unhedged care. We feel emotionally vulnerable, our hearts dangerously unguarded against the pain we might experience at the hands of whatever disaster may befall us. But the fact of the matter is that no matter what disaster may befall us, our preemptive concern over it does not mitigate the heartache it will cause in the least. Nor was any true disaster ever averted by worry. All worry does, in fact, is rob us of present care and love and enjoyment by pulling our thoughts into a negative, fearful future.

HOW TO BUILD A WORKOUT USING A SIMPLE "300"-INSPIRED PROTOCOL

Originally published on SuperheroSimplified.blogspot.com
February 3, 2014

People come to my Strength & Conditioning classes for a variety of reasons. Some people like the group atmosphere, some need a coach to motivate them, some like the variety of strange new implements. Some people are there because they know that exercise is important (even if they don't quite know why), while others are athletes looking to improve their performance in their chosen sport. There are others, however, who come to me for a more basic reason: they have the desire to work out, the willingness to invest their energy, but they have no idea how to compose a workout.

Maybe they spent their high school and college athletic years in weight rooms with coaches and teammates guiding them through sport-specific or equipment-specific protocols. Maybe they didn't play sports, and have no idea where to start. Or maybe they simply feel overwhelmed or frustrated by the mountain of (often contradictory) information available to them on YouTube, in fitness magazines, in "Behind the Fight" TV specials, etc.

These people often end up as runners. They think, "I need to get back in shape," and running seems like the safest bet. You can't go wrong with running, right? And running is the best form of exercise, right? (Didn't I read that somewhere, maybe in a running magazine?)

This post is not the time or place for me to list the reasons I think running (or at least the way people in this fitness culture run) is a misguided waste of time. Suffice it to say, for now, that: 1) long-phase steady-pace cardiovascular activity has been shown to make you fatter, 2) running (or, again, the way most people run) beats up your knees, hips, and lower back, and 3) running does not promote a general state of functional fitness (meaning that running does not produce functional strength and endurance for anything except running).

Ask any of my runner friends, and they will tell you that my attitude is: If you love running, then by all means run. If you don't love running—if you're only running because you literally can't think of anything better to do (if you can't come up with another way to work yourself out)—then this post is for you.

You may have read my previous post *Castaway Fitness*, in which I outline some basic protocols for composing a well-rounded functional workout. If you haven't, there's a lot of good information in that post along these same lines. In that post I organized working out around major movement patterns (again, look back at that article if you don't know what I'm talking about), but I'm going to make this post even more basic (read: accessible). In this post I'm going to tell you how to compose a great workout that will give you more benefit than a run, and take far less time, inspired by the protocol used when training the actors for the movie *300*.

The original 300 workout was a challenge set up by Mark Twight and his team at Gym Jones in Salt Lake City, UT. It consisted of varied sets of a handful of exercises which had to be performed in less than 15 minutes. After the movie came out, and America saw Gerard Butler's abs, everyone and their mother jumped on the *300* bandwagon, promising ridiculous results with their own version of the 300 workout.

Then America—like it always does—realized that working out is hard, that results aren't magically instant, and the 300 workout fell by the wayside.

I like the idea behind the 300 protocol, and I've made many 300-inspired workouts, and they've all kicked my butt. I also think it's a fantastically easy way to compose a workout if you're not a fitness professional, but just someone trying to get a workout in while you're away from home or away from your home gym.

The original 300 workout included varied sets and a single cycle through the circuit. For ease and variety, I use a 10/10/3x arrangement: 10 repetitions of each of 10 exercises, cycled through 3 times for 300 total repetitions, done in 15 minutes or less.

So to build your own 300 workout, simply make a list of 10 of your favorite (or least favorite) exercises. These can be equipment-specific or bodyweight, depending on what you have available to you. The variety of exercises will give you a fantastic muscular demand, while the pace you have to keep in order to meet the 15 minute limit will tax your cardiovascular capacity like you wouldn't believe.

As a reference, here's a list of some basic exercises you could incorporate into your 300 workout.

Bodyweight exercises: push-up, pull-up, bodyweight row, squat, jumping from a squat, jumping from a squat and pulling your knees up into your chest at the top of the jump, burpee (sprawl out into a plank, hop back up to your feet, and jump), deck squat, stepping lunge, plyometric lunge, sprawl, Hindu push-up, bodyweight dip, etc.

Equipment-specific exercises: dead lift, clean, hang clean, clean and jerk, clean and press, kettlebell swing, weighted squat, kettlebell clean, kettlebell deck squat, kettlebell halo, etc.

So, drawing on this list, we might make a workout that looks like this:

1. Push-up

2. Jump from a low squat
3. Pull-up
4. Kettlebell swing
5. Burpee
6. Bodyweight dip
7. Kettlebell halo (10R, 10L)
8. Bodyweight row
9. Dead lift
10. Sprawl

10 reps of each exercise, 3 times through, in 15 minutes or less.

Give the 300 protocol a try the next time you're at a loss for how to compose a workout, or the next time you're looking out the window at Cleveland in mid-February and your running shoes just somehow aren't making their way onto your feet.

Stay super!

THE SUPERHERO SIMPLIFIED TRIPLE AUGHT (ORDER OF OPERATIONS)

Originally published on SuperheroSimplified.blogspot.com
February 10, 2014

Embarking on a new diet is a commendable undertaking. As with most things, the hardest step is the first one, and once you've made the commitment to getting your diet in order—no matter what dietary philosophy you follow—you are on the right track, and I salute you.

Unfortunately, the second hardest step is often the step *back* onto the right track. Our dietary efforts can get derailed in a million ways, and one misstep too often opens the door to others (as in: "Well, my diet is already shot for today anyway..."). Making things more difficult, the decision to step back onto the right track is argued against the voice of a new enemy: real world experience. After all, in the beginning, the NEW DIET was all daydreams and rainbows: it promised easy lifestyle modifications and nearly effortless (and dramatic) results. But one or two or ten or twenty days in we know the truth: those lifestyle modifications aren't so easy and those results are often far from dramatic. Faced with the task of recommitting, we may find doubt or frustration in place of hope and resolve, and may allow these to torpedo the whole endeavor.

Thus the beneficial and commendable core impulse (the golden nugget of good intentions, the will to change and get healthy) which started us down this path gets thrown out along with the faulty execution (the NEW DIET that failed).

Diets (the kind you "go on," not the kind you live with) fail for all sorts of reasons, but seem to most often fail because they're simply unlivable. You've heard it before, but I'll say it again: a successful diet is all about sustainable behavior. Yes you can technically survive on broth, and you will lose weight, but let's face it: you *won't* survive on broth. Not if you're not forced to. Neither will I. Neither will anyone in their right mind. Sooner or later our willpower breaks down. Not because we're weak necessarily, but rather because we created a condition that we couldn't reasonably expect ourselves to endure or sustain. I think too often the unsustainable nature of a NEW DIET doesn't deter adherents because culturally we understand "dieting" to be a massive but limited-term undertaking, the equivalent of being on your "best behavior" until a deadline (the weight loss goal, or a wedding, or a high school reunion) is reached. But in this approach the long-term impact or health benefit of this approach is disregarded, and even the short-term health impact can often be disregarded, superseded in the eyes of the adherent by the *appearance* of a *symptom* (body fat loss) rather than a true environmental (the health of the body in sum) shift.

If short-term superficial change is the extent of your goal, then more power to you. But I have a suggestion: If you're looking for an easy way to lose weight, and you don't care whether or not it's good for you, go hang around a hospital until you catch the flu. You'll drop a dress size in no time flat.

A healthy diet is about health, not about weight loss. A healthy body with a healthy hormone profile does not store or carry excess body fat. Weight loss is a product of health (just as excess body fat is a symptom of an unhealthy condition), but a diet focused on weight loss alone will often pursue unsustainable (and often downright unhealthy) tactics. The flu is a great way to lose superficial weight, but that doesn't make it healthy.

As I said in the beginning of this post, the commitment to improving one's health is a commendable undertaking, and if you've made that commitment then I want to do all I can to help you avoid some of the common pitfalls (massive and immediate lifestyle changes, hunger, lack of results) and make your transition a successful one. So what follows is what I like to call the Superhero Simplified Triple Aught: the Order of Operations for integrating a new diet into your life (not the life you pretend to live for a couple months leading up to beach season).

Follow this order of operations one step at a time. Move onto the next step only after you've implemented the previous step and acclimated to your new dietary habits (i.e. made them your new normal). This can mean spending weeks or even months on each step. This is a marathon, not a sprint. And bear in mind that you didn't put all the weight on in a week, and you're not going to take it off in a week, either.

Operation # 1: Cut out refined sugar.

This is going to be harder than it sounds, but I believe in you. Refined sugar, in this case, means any plant sugar that has been removed from its fibrous plant environment. This includes white sugar, high fructose corn syrup, cane sugar, agave nectar, maple syrup, and the lot. The simple reason here is that sugar ingested in a rapidly digestible form is pretty doggone bad for you, and is responsible for your insulin dump "food comas" and that last ten pounds that seems so resistant to your eviction efforts. Simple carbohydrates that you don't burn off more or less immediately get stored.

Operation # 2: Cut out wheat, corn, and rice.

Ok, hold your horses, I know this is practically a political state-ment. I'm not trying to push an agenda beyond saying: this has worked wonders for me, and has worked wonders for everyone I've counseled who has actually implemented it. I don't even need you to believe that wheat or corn or rice are bad for you (there is plenty of evidence in both camps). What I am going to suggest is that many of us subsist on a diet based too heavily on these easily accessible fuels, and these fuels get stored as body fat when they don't get used up. And yes, there is an argument to be had here about calories ingested/ calories burned (i.e. Can't I just keep eating bread and run more?) but why bother having it? If you're only running to burn off the carbs, then why not skip (or at least drastically reduce) the carbs? Again, I know people are going to argue with me on this one, but just think about it for a minute: corn, wheat, and rice are bases. They're filler. In most dishes in most restaurants, they *hold* the food that you actually want to eat. Do you really care that much about rice? Do you care that much about the bun on your hamburger? What is a tortilla but an edible utensil?

This seems like a good time for a note about the "calories ingest-ed/calories burned" model of dieting. For the record, this model seems to be at the very least incomplete, if not outright wrong. As I said, a healthy body does not store excess body fat because to do so would be detrimental to its function. However, it is possible to over-ride your body's desire to shed by constantly feeding it more fuel to store. Again, whether you believe me or not, I think this step is easier than you think, and you have nothing to lose by trying it (except the weight). And, if you really love the notion of calories ingested/calo-ries burned, then just try thinking of it instead as: carbs ingested/ carbs burned.

Operation # 3: Cut out snacks.

Really we're getting down to the nitty gritty, because I think if you follow the last two operations for any length of time you're going to find your weight loss goals pretty close at hand. This step is about health as much as it is about weight loss: digestion is work, and work is stress, and if you are eating every hour or so then your body is constantly working to digest food. That can start to drag on your system. Leaving a break between meals benefits your health by giving your digestive tract a chance to rest and repair itself. And by cutting out snacks, I mean leave 4 or so hours between meals. I'm not suggesting major periods of deprivation. If you're not feeling blood sugar dips (often confused for hunger, and related to a diet based on the foods we cut out in operations 1 and 2) I think you're going to find that this isn't much of an issue.

Operation # 4: Stick to single ingredient foods.

I think the logic behind this one is pretty self-evident, but let me illustrate using the following story. When I was three, I swallowed a marble. Everyone was worried, but then the next day the marble came out and there was no harm done. When we eat food out of a box, a lot of the time we're eating marbles. We can't digest some of the ingredients, and we don't really know what they are, and they don't nourish us, but they don't seem to be killing us. So could you keep doing it? Who knows? But either way, how long do you want to keep eating marbles? Think of it this way: you eat food so you have energy to work to make money so you can buy food... that doesn't really give you energy? Think about it. Stop eating marbles.

Operation # 5: Work out.

What? Wait this long? But I always thought working out was the most important thing! Eh. Not so much. I mostly put this step this far down the list to let you know just how unimportant I think working out is to weight loss. This doesn't mean don't work out—if you enjoy working out then by all means do it. What it does mean, however, is don't work out thinking that what you do in the gym is going to be the final word—or even the majority word—in your weight loss efforts. The big problem we see today is people with poor diets (and in less than optimum health) starting aggressive workout programs thinking that this will improve their health and fitness. Often it has the opposite effect: a body overtaxed by the detrimental effects of a poor diet is further burdened with the stress of aggressive training, and is made *less* healthy in the process. Have a friend who runs five to eight miles every morning, loves cupcakes, and has a cold they just can't kick? Then you already know what I'm talking about.

Implement these steps over the course of six months, even a year. Feel comfortable at each step before you move on to the next step. If you fall off track, you've only fallen off one track. Ate some refined sugar? No big deal—the next time you put something in your mouth, make sure it's something without refined sugar. You haven't ruined the whole thing. Remember that every bite you take is a vote for what kind of body you want.

Keep at it. And cheers to you for making the effort.

Until next time, stay super.

WHAT (AND HOW) SUPER SCOTT EATS IN HIS DAY-TO-DAY LIFE

Originally published on SuperheroSimplified.blogspot.com
February 17, 2014

I've got a few people in my orbit looking to make some dietary changes (good on ya, gents!), and hitting a bit of a snag: they know the foods they want to avoid, they know why they want to avoid them, but what they haven't been able to do is come up with a new dietary pattern to replace the old one—to come up with a new regular roster of meals and snacks that will both satisfy their hunger and (after the initial adjustment) consume a comparable amount of time and energy in preparation to their former roster of dietary regulars. This post, then, is to help you guys (and anyone else out there looking to change their diet) integrate dietary principles into dietary behaviors.

First, a quick rundown of the principles. What do I eat? I tend to describe my diet in a couple of different ways: sometimes I say that I eat "plants and animals." Other times I say that, "If it didn't come out of the ground or have a mother, I don't eat it." Basically I eat meat, cultured (full fat) dairy (cheese, yogurt, and kefir), vegetables, nuts, and fruit. I avoid what I call the "five white foods": sugar, wheat, rice, corn, and white potatoes (listed in most aggressively avoided to least).

Now the hangup that a lot of people hit: they think, "Man, I have to apply these rules to every possible meal I'm going to eat for the rest of my life? I'll never manage that!" I'll admit that, when you look at it that way, the task does seem daunting. But, if you think about it for a minute, and if you're anything like me, I think you'll discover that your roster of regular meals and snacks is fairly limited. Don't you eat one of maybe four or five different "snack foods" every day? Don't you eat the same thing for breakfast ninety-five percent of the time? Your family may even have a regular weekly schedule of meals.

For my Sidekick/Partner in Crime and I, the key to changing our diet wasn't in coming up with a healthy version of every possible meal we would ever eat forever, or even in finding a new meal to entirely replace an old, unhealthy standard. In the beginning, the key was finding a healthier meal to replace each of our standard roster meals (remember that in this case "healthier" doesn't mean flavorless, fatless, or even less). Later, we worked in new recipes, and even found new regulars that we liked even better than old ones, but in the beginning it was just a matter of getting the pizza and the pasta and the fish sticks and french fries out of our lives in such a way that we wouldn't even miss them.

As you're maybe starting to see, the basic principle (eat only plants and animals, avoid the big five) is pretty easy to apply to pretty much any meal, anywhere. For illustration, here are some home- and restaurant-friendly ideas, with their "typical" counterparts.

BREAKFAST

Typical: Eggs/Bacon/Hash browns/Toast
Modified: Eggs/Bacon/Avocado or Tomato slices/Cottage Cheese

Typical: Low-fat milk and cereal
Modified: Full-fat Greek yogurt with almonds or cashews and fruit.

Or just a fruit meal is awesome in the morning, like melon or something citrus. I avoid fruit juices for the same reason I avoid refined sugar: without the fibrous pulp, that fruit sugar dumps right into your bloodstream.

Sometimes I'll do a sliced apple with cream cheese. Way better than a bagel and cream cheese.

LUNCH

Typical: Sandwich with chips
Modified: Lunch meat and cheese from the deli counter, eaten rolled up with spinach in the middle. This meal will remind you that the bread is pretty much just there to hold everything together. You won't miss it.

Typical: Hamburger with french fries.
Modified: Hamburger patty on a bed of lettuce/salad. Pile on the tomatoes, onions, cheese, pickles. I steer clear of ketchup: there's added sugar hiding in there.

Another of my go-to lunches is a pile of cottage cheese with almonds and fruit. Or some sliced cheese and a couple of apples or pears.

DINNER

Typical: Pizza
Modified: Chicken parmesan. Same cheesy, oregano-y, marinara-y goodness, but on chicken. I make my own marinara, because a lot of store-bought stuff has added sugar (it's everywhere) but even if you don't go that far, just making the switch (and dumping the crust) is a fantastic start

Typical: Tacos

Modified: Taco salad. Cook up some ground beef or chicken (we usually do chicken) with some onions, slice up some tomatoes, make some guacamole, get some salsa, shred some cheese, eat it all on a bed of shredded lettuce... Nothing to miss except the annoyance of having your shells break and spill into your lap.

Typical: Pot roast with mashed potatoes.

Modified: Ever tried mashed cauliflower? I think it's actually better than mashed potatoes, and neatly avoids the starch bomb. That's a simple swap. Enjoy. The same modification can be made to shepherd's pie, turkey dinner, etc.

SNACKS

This one is the killer, isn't it? Granola bars, crackers, cookies, pretzels, chips... The list goes on and on.

Here's the thing about snacks. A lot of the time, we're not eating them because we're hungry. We're eating them because 1) they're there, and 2) our blood sugar is crashing, because the last thing we ate was heavy on one of the big five. So once you eliminate the big five (especially the first one, sugar), and you get over the "detox" phase (sugar is a drug, expect a detox phase), don't be surprised if you find yourself "hungry" (aka blood sugar crashing) less often. (Also, obviously, not having that stuff in your house is the easiest way to deal with the first thing.)

Now, after that, you may find that you are snacking because you are hungry. And the question is: Are you hungry because you didn't eat to satisfaction at your last meal? And the question then is: Why not? Snacking may or may not be a bad habit (there's debate) but one thing is clear: if you eat until you're full, you're full. So focus on eating meals composed of good elements until you don't want any more, and you may also find that this curbs your snack habit.

But if you still want to snack, I recommend going with small portions of some of the go-to lunches and breakfasts I listed above: an apple and some cream cheese, cottage cheese and fruit, some deli meat and cheese, some fruit and nuts. These are my go-to choices now and, just like before, when I would hit the snack aisle at two o'clock, I go to the produce or the dairy section without thinking about it.

As I think you can maybe see, a lot of what I eat is the same as what you eat... with maybe one or two degrees of difference. These changes are easy to make, and well worth the effort.

So good for you for deciding you want to make this change. Keep at it. In six months, these decisions will be habits, and you won't even think about them.

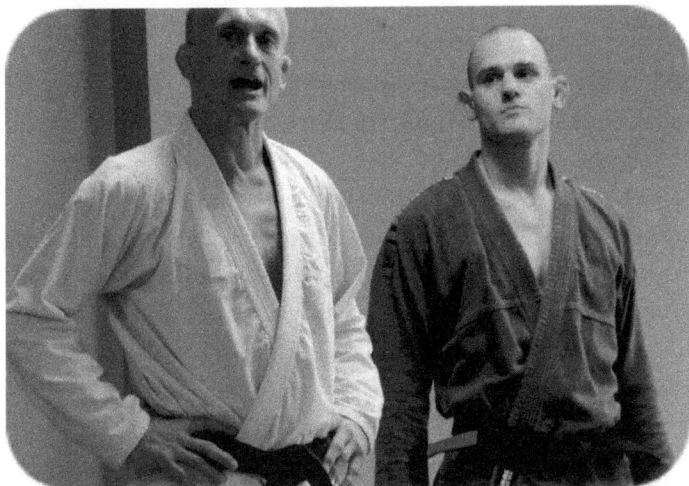

FAIXA PRETA

Originally published on SuperheroSimplified.blogspot.com
April 14, 2014

In the martial arts, when someone gets promoted, only they get to wear the new belt. The accolades don't get spread around. Only one guy gets congratulated.

I got promoted to black belt yesterday. It's been a longtime goal of mine. I got to stand up in front of everybody and have that coveted belt tied around my waist. It meant and means a lot to me. I don't know that trying to put it into words will add anything to this. Those of you who get it already get it.

Of the American fantastical archetypes, there's one we seem to adore above all others: the self-made man, the self-reliant hero, the rugged individualist. We love loners and cooly competent Armies of one. We love Hemingway and Teddy Roosevelt and MacGyver. Just try and tell me you wouldn't rather see Batman without Robin.

The fallacy at the core of this myth, the far-reaching and damaging effects of this archetype, are a bigger subject, and one for another post. Right now, all I want to say is that, as much as we may like these characters, and may wish to feel that special kind of stoic pride and final, unmitigated admirability, none of us get where we are by our efforts alone. None of us take full credit for our accomplishments.

One of the things I love about Brazilian Jiu-Jitsu is the way it joins people together. You find a kind of community in a lot of BJJ gyms that you just don't see most other places (at least I haven't found it). Words like "brotherhood" and "family" get thrown around a lot, and are maybe overused and abused, but I still think it's fair to say that what happens on the mat comes to more than the loose affiliation of strangers you find in most "communities" these days.

Which is why, as much as I'd like to accept this promotion, I just can't.

I can't because—frankly—it's not mine to accept. At least it's not all mine. The better part of it belongs to everyone I've trained and sweated and (not to be dramatic, but it is technically correct) bled with. *I* didn't make me good enough to deserve this promotion. *You guys* made me good enough. You guys pushed me and challenged me and taught me and supported me. You guys (Jason) believed in me and gave me a place to work and teach and let me spend my time training. You guys (Steve) gave me more of your time and knowledge and insight than I had any right to expect. You guys (Jen) didn't complain when I ran off for hours on our vacations to train at other gyms. You guys came to the gym and thought enough of my teaching to pay me so that I could pay my rent and didn't have to get some other job that would take me away from Jiu-Jitsu.

So I can't really accept whatever portion of this achievement I can claim as my own without also giving credit to those who share it.

To my teachers, thank you. Steve, having the opportunity to learn from you has been a completely undeserved gift. Jason, you've done more for me than pretty much anyone, and you've always acted like it's no big deal. But it is a big deal. I can't thank you enough. Darren, you've given me so much of your time and energy. All of you have shown me so much generosity. I am profoundly grateful to you all.

To all of my students and training partners: for beating me up, for getting beat up, for asking me questions and making me really know what I'm talking about: Thank you. One of the great truths of BJJ is that you only get as good as your training partners make you get. Any progress I've made I owe to you. Thank you.

To my mother, for supporting me and encouraging me and affirming my endeavors, though they are almost a complete waste of a really expensive college education, and for reminding me that my ears used to be cute: Thank you.

To Jen, for understanding when I spent a big chunk of our (limited) time in New York or Florida or wherever rolling around on the floor with a bunch of strangers in pajamas, and for being my partner in crime. Thank you.

I am so profoundly grateful to each of you who took part of your own life—your time, your energy, your knowledge—and expended it on me. Thank you, thank you, thank you. Whatever is good or exciting or laudable in this promotion belongs to you.

ACUTE PROBLEMS GET SOLVED

Originally published on SuperheroSimplified.blogspot.com
April 21, 2014

We all have problems, issues, things we'd like to change about ourselves and our lives. Sometimes these problems rear up and demand our attention, but more often they simmer along quietly in the background, avoiding resolution. Sometimes these simmering problems can simmer for weeks, months, even years.

Maybe you've been meaning to go on a diet. Maybe you've been meaning to start working out. Maybe you've been meaning to spend more time with your family, to work on your relationship with your spouse or your kids. Maybe you've been thinking about quitting your job, and doing something else with your life. Maybe you've been telling yourself that pretty soon—when things lighten up at work or when the holidays are over or when this situation with your company's merger resolves itself or when you've paid off the mortgage—you'll get to it.

Among our other amazing faculties, human beings possess an absolutely staggering ability to adapt to our circumstances. Look at the way people have lived and still live in extreme and harrowing conditions. Look at the way we manage calamities and disasters, at the way we conform and innovate. We have a seemingly endless capacity for normalization, for reorienting ourselves and our perceptions to our surroundings. Even bizarre alterations to our lives quickly become our new normal.

But "new normal" can become a trap. In the same way that people learn to live with the loss of a limb or rapidly altered financial circumstances, we quickly integrate simmering problems into our perception of "normal," and pretty soon these simmering problems—these "I'll get to it as soon as _____ is resolved" problems—become no longer problems we plan to one day fix, but rather ongoing conditions of our lives. We know we need to get back in shape. We know we need to change our diets. We know we need to spend more time with our families. We know we need to find new jobs. We know we need to fix any one of a hundred things that make our daily lives a place we don't like and don't want to be, but somehow we don't. Instead we bitch about our jobs and we watch sports and we drink beer and we anesthetize ourselves with mindlessness. We buy things because they promise that in owning them we will magically also possess a life that's radically different from our own, a life in which we're no longer plagued by these chronic problems. And we keep on telling ourselves that someday, as soon as _____, we'll get around to doing all those things we know we need to do.

And time goes by, and we get older and older and older.

The problem with "someday" is that it rarely comes. A person in motion tends to stay in motion, down the same track they've been running on, and pretty soon what I'm doing right now, just until _____, becomes what I've been doing for a month and a year and five years and ten years and my entire life.

Except when something bad happens. Then things change. The problems that rear up and demand your immediate response can jar you off that track. Tragedy strikes or the bottom falls out of the market or someone close to you develops a life-altering addiction. Someone in your family gets sick. Somebody wrecks a car.

You solve those problems. Until they're resolved those problems become your whole life. Nothing can resume until those problems are fixed. Changes are made, and your life is not quite the same afterwards.

The simple fact of the matter is that most of us are incapable of making a sustained change by sheer force of will. The gravity of complacency is just too strong. We need disasters—acute, immediate problems—to jar us out of normalcy. But this is not necessarily a question of the extremity or the urgency of the problem: this can be a question of my *perception* of the problem. If my weight or my job becomes an intolerable situation by my deciding that it is, then I will not be content to allow my life to continue as is. If, every time I see myself in a mirror, or sit through a boring meeting, or wake up early on Monday hating my life, I allow myself to feel the immediate and acute sting of dissatisfaction—and if I reinforce that perception with every subsequent interaction with that problem, and perceive my efforts in the resolution of that problem as tangible steps toward the resolution of that problem (regardless of external indicator)—then I will take steps and will continue to take steps to solve that problem.

If that seems overly simple, let me give you an example to illustrate how this might work.

Joe has been steadily gaining weight since his late twenties. Now he's thirty-five, and is twenty pounds overweight. He put the weight on slowly, and now it's just what he's used to looking like. All of his clothes fit his current body. All of the pictures he sees of himself on Facebook show him looking the way he looks now. He is vaguely aware that he doesn't love the way he looks (or feels), but most of the time he doesn't think about it. He's only acutely aware of it once in a while—when he goes to the doctor's office, when he goes on a date, when he eats something really bad. The rest of the time it's just in the background. He doesn't look in the mirror when he's getting into the shower, and the mirror is too fogged up to show his reflection by the time he gets out.

On top of this, Joe's friends all look like him. They're about twenty pounds overweight. One of his friends is forty pounds overweight and, even though none of them would ever say it, the heaviest friend's presence makes them all feel a little better about themselves. It makes them feel like, all things considered, they aren't really in that bad a shape. At least not as bad as that guy.

Joe takes an ironic, sarcastic stance toward "bros" who hang out in the gym all day. He and his friends make jokes about how out of shape they themselves are: how they would die if they ever tried to run a marathon, etc. Whatever acute self-consciousness he feels is glossed over with a weak attempt at humor and then shoved to the back of his mind in the file along with awkward first kisses and the time he got pantsed at recess in the fourth grade: along with all of the other things he doesn't want to think about.

Joe's weight problem is chronic, and because it is chronic it is also timeless. He knows he needs to work out more, to change what he eats, but he just doesn't have the time or the energy right now. There's no room in his life for that, no framework in place. When would he go to the gym? And how could he justify ordering a salad when everyone else is ordering fries? Think of the grief they would give him!

Joe vaguely imagines that maybe over the summer, when the weather's better, he'll start running. He imagines making a New Year's resolution this year, and sticking with it. But New Year's is months away, and after it finally arrives he's too busy catching up with the work he let slide over the holidays to start running, too tired to make a change.

Or imagine this: Joe wakes up one morning and he looks in the mirror and he sees that extra weight around his middle and under his chin like it's a spider or a cobweb or a leech, something that he wants off of him *right now*. He allows himself to feel, for fifteen or thirty seconds, the visceral immediacy of this problem. He has no trouble tying on his running shoes, now. He has no trouble skipping those donuts in the break room. There's something unbearable ON HIM, and he wants it off. And every step Joe takes, every donut he doesn't eat, he sees as another hammer strike against the problem, another dent in the wall, another step toward his goal. It's an act of faith at first, but pretty soon he starts to see the evidence of his work, and he doesn't have to tell himself that these steps are working because it's obvious that they are.

Chronic problems go in the bucket of problems I'll solve "someday." Acute problems get solved today, this week, this month, *right f*cking now*. The difference between a chronic problem and an acute one doesn't *have* to be dramatic. A tree doesn't *have* to fall on your house. You *don't* have to get diagnosed with a disease (in fact, you hear stories all the time about people for whom even a disease diagnosis isn't acute enough: diabetics who don't change their diets, lung cancer patients who don't stop smoking, etc.). The difference between acute and chronic can be *your decision*. Make your problems intolerable by deciding that you can't tolerate them anymore. Decide that these circumstances are unacceptable.

Your time is the single most precious thing you have: don't waste any more of it living in a way you aren't satisfied with. Don't let more hours slip away from you waiting for the "someday" when you're going to actualize your ideal self. That "someday" is either today, or it's never. Do it right *now*.

I HOPE YOU'RE PROUD OF YOURSELF

Originally published on SuperheroSimplified.blogspot.com
April 28, 2014

I am part of the self-esteem generation. When I was growing up, the predominant theory being advanced by experts in child-rearing was that a child's self-esteem was the key to his or her success and happiness. Among other things, this theory helped to produce the much-ballyhooed "everyone gets a trophy" phenomenon, the entitlement at the core of the "snowflake" theory of personality, the "big is beautiful" self-image campaign, and a host of other, in the long run, detrimental social stances that we're now trying to pull ourselves out of.

In the abstract, everyone does have the right to feel good about themselves. Everyone has the right to be proud of themselves, and of their bodies. But bodies and selves aren't abstractions: they're aggregates of our past behaviors. Your "self"—the person you imagine when you think of yourself, and the person we think of when we think of you—is largely a question of what you've done. What kind of person have you shown yourself to be by your actions? Have you performed the acts of the person you want to be? Have you performed acts that make you proud? Similarly, your body is not just the product of your genetics. Certainly some people carry more muscle mass and less body fat; some people are taller than others, some are shorter, etc. But within the parameters of your physical potential, your body is the product of your behaviors.

Out drinking every night? Finding any excuse for a sugary coffee, or an ice cream? Nibbling cookies every day at lunch? Look in the mirror: Your behavior is showing.

I don't want to tell anyone to feel bad about themselves, or about how they look. I am saying, however, that the idea of being "proud" of one's self or one's body is ridiculous if that self or that body is the product of behaviors of which you are not and should not and cannot be proud.

You can look elsewhere on this blog and find my personal take on diet, on which foods I think you're better off cutting out of your life, on how much exercise you should be getting, etc. I don't want to get into a big thing here about how you should be behaving. And for the most part, I don't think I really need to. I'm not talking about whether or not you stuck to your new firehouse paleo vegan upside-down handstand diet one hundred percent. I'm not talking about only being proud of yourself when you're perfect. I'm talking about the really basic basics: you know cookies aren't good for you. You know that microwaved gas station burrito wasn't the best meal choice you ever made. You know that Big Mac didn't do you any favors. I'm talking about the moments when you slipped your mental police officer a five and told him to look the other way for a minute. I'm talking about the times when you knew better, and you did it anyway.

There is a longer blog post coming sooner or later about what I feel to be the net increase in hopelessness engendered by the concept of the eternal self, but for now all I want to point out is that the really incredible notion at the core of this post is that the self and the body and the ways we feel about them are not the ethereal prison they can sometimes seem to be. You are not innately the way you feel about yourself today, good or bad. Nor are you innately—no matter how many diets have failed you—the way you look. You build yourself and your body every day with every meaningful action you take: If you did something you're not proud of yesterday—if you lost your temper and kicked the dog or you ate cake for breakfast—you have another chance in every subsequent second of your life to do something of which you are proud.

So skip the cupcake. Go to the gym. When your jeans fit well, be proud of that. When they don't—when you've made some of those not-so-admirable choices—nothing in the world is going to make you feel better except doing something of which you can be proud. You can't buy a new outfit and have that bad feeling go away. You can't talk your way out of it. You can't tell the world that you have a right to feel good about your doughy midsection. If you look in the mirror and feel bad, it's your behavior you're feeling bad about. You want to feel better? Behave better. Then you'll look better. Then you'll feel better.

I feel like I need to also point out that this isn't a question of other people judging you. This isn't a question of an unrealistic cultural standard of beauty. This isn't a question of you having more value as a person if you're good-looking. It is a question of how you feel about yourself. I'm not talking about being tall, dark, and handsome. I'm not talking about symmetrical features or action figure biceps. I'm talking about your double chin and your spare tire and the bags under your eyes. I'm talking about the physical manifestations of your behavior. Lose those and, despite your lack of symmetrical features and all the rest of it, you'll be surprised how beautiful healthy looks.

Start right now. Build a self, a body, a life you can be proud of. Build it one commendable act at a time. Because you do have the right to feel good about yourself.

IGNORANCE IS BLISS

Originally published on SuperheroSimplified.blogspot.com
May 5, 2014

There's an important distinction that often gets lost in our crazy, mixed-up world.

Ignorance is not knowing something because you've never been taught it. I am ignorant of the cultural customs of the native peoples of Papua New Guinea, etc.

Stupidity is not knowing something because, despite having been exposed to it, you choose to ignore the information with which you've been presented in favor of your own, prior, ignorant understanding.

Ignorance isn't your fault. We're all ignorant of what we haven't learned. The world is full of things that any one individual doesn't understand, and will likely never learn. The world is big and life is short and mysteries abound.

Stupidity, however, *is* your fault, because to be stupid, you must *choose* to be ignorant.

You might be asking yourself why anyone in their right mind would ever choose to be ignorant. It doesn't make sense and yet, if you take a second to think about it, I think you'll find that we make this subtle choice all the time.

Have you ever been grappling with a problem and had someone come up and, after a cursory examination, suggest a solution you hadn't considered? Have you ever, in annoyance, dismissed them and their idea, though you know it's better? Have you continued with your approach just to spite them, because you want them to be wrong?

Ever been drawn into an argument with someone who clearly knows more than you about the subject of the argument? Ever categorically rejected their point of view for reasons having nothing to do with the subject at hand (the "I'm right because that guy's a jerk" approach to debate)?

Ever had a doctor tell you that you need to change your diet, and exercise more? Ever had dessert at the next meal anyway?

And in every instance: Have you ever reassured yourself that the other party didn't really understand, for one reason or another, and that you (of course) retain the right to be the final authority in your own little experience?

I definitely have. I think maybe you have, too. We all do. We choose—very subtly, and without really looking it in the eye—to ignore the better information. We know better, yet we allow our irrational, emotional side to steer us.

We do this for any number of reasons. Maybe when someone confronts us with what we don't know we feel threatened (maybe rightfully so; maybe this person is very clearly trying to "knock us down a peg" by demonstrating their superior knowledge or skill, and trying to up their own social standing by demonstrating this superiority in front of our peers). Maybe we made a decision based on an assumption a long time ago, and now we feel we've gone too far to start over. Or maybe we reject it simply because the information itself implies our ignorance—implies the limit of our knowledge or understanding or capability—and the appearance of this naked limit is itself threatening.

Whatever the reason, we reject better, more useful information in favor of the illusion of our own autonomous and unimpeachable and unified authority. But of course the problem with this approach—with choosing to remain ignorant—is that we become, in effect, stupid.

When we're confronted with our own ignorance, the decision we have to make is the following: Will I admit to myself and to whoever is watching that I don't know, that my ideas are unsound, that I am ignorant, and in so doing open myself up to learning something new, a better approach, etc., or would I rather keep knowing what I know, and be stupid? These really are the only two options available. And, as you may notice, being stupid doesn't make you less ignorant. It just prolongs your time living there.

If those sound like two bad options, then you're seriously under-estimating how amazing ignorance is. When you forgo the burden of being the final authority in your own little world, when you realize that your ignorance is no threat to you, that it in no way diminishes your value as a person to not know what you don't know, then you can open your eyes without hesitation or fear to the universe of subjects and knowledge and undertakings you've previously eschewed, avoided, run from, hidden from.

Try it. Consider the possibility that someone else is right and that you should do what he or she says and think what he or she thinks. Let go of your silly simian need to see yourself as living at the top of your own imaginary hierarchy. There's a whole world out there, lying just beyond the borders of what you think you understand. So do the smart thing. Stop being stupid, and embrace your ignorance.

DRY LAND IS A MYTH

Originally published on SuperheroSimplified.blogspot.com
May 26, 2014

Whatever else you can say about Kevin Costner's 1995 box office disaster *Waterworld*, it still managed to strike on one unimpeachable truth: Dry land is a myth.

Don't worry, this isn't a post about climate change and melting polar ice caps. This post is about the economics of energy (and again: no, I don't mean energy from fossil fuels). I mean the economics of vital energy: of time and attention and patience and effort.

It is in our nature to form networks of social interaction. We do it at work, at the gym, at church, at our regular coffee shop, at the mall. We mentally log faces and locations and contexts. Sometimes these relationships grow into friendships, more often they don't. Sometimes these relationships grow into romances, more often they don't. Whether they grow into something more or remain casual, however, these relationships always develop their own particular parameters.

This is the nature of social interaction. Person A says something general to Person B, and offers a general opinion about it ("It is so nice that summer is finally here."). Person B replies with a similar statement ("I know! I was getting so sick of winter."). The conversation can remain at this level, or delve deeper: Person A offers something more specific ("My kids love the snow, but even they were like, enough already!"); Person B responds in kind, or encourages Person A ("I know, my kids are so sick of being cooped up inside/How old are your kids?"). Etc., etc. The conversation continues or it doesn't continue, each person divulging more information specific to themselves as individuals, or not.

These interactions become part of the vast store of information that we, as social animals, catalog and track. We may not remember the details shared, but we do tend to remember the depth of the conversation: how "far" we let someone into our private minds. We log dozens and dozens of bits of situation-specific information about these interactions.

All right, so what does this have to do with dry land?

Just as we, in our search for connection, move through these interactions searching for the parameters of the meeting (i.e. will this offering of personal information be returned in kind, or rebuffed?), so too we must bear in mind that our counterpart is searching for parameters: that they are asking us, in effect, what sort of offering or behavior or divulgence is allowed in this relationship. More often than not our parameters are not tested: rarely are we met with someone who forces us to decide whether to allow something into the exchange. Sometimes, however, we end up cornered by an interpersonal boundary pusher.

I'm not talking about gross imposition, crass behavior, or generally inappropriate offerings (these are all—despite and, in fact, because of their extremity—easy enough to handle: a rude joke or a racist comment easily stirs us to conversational action, bolstered by the self-assurance that society agrees with my taking offense). I'm talking about the slight imposition, the slight request, the conversational nudge, the verbal drag that edges its way past acceptable so gently and stealthily that soon, without knowing how we arrived there, we are in unpleasant territory.

Think about the waitress who shares a bit too much about how hard a time she's having in nursing school. Think about the opposite-sex stranger who starts telling you too much about how their marriage is in trouble. Think about the sibling who divulges too much about their money issues, or the coworker who always tells you all about their problem child. Think about your significant other, who guilts you when you go to the gym. Or the hairdresser who is having car trouble. Or the friend who makes endless sexist comments. Each of these interactions started somewhere normal and acceptable, and then veered wildly off course. In each we had a chance to exert authority over our own conversational or interpersonal parameters (what sort of offerings we would and would not accept) and yet, either because we were "too nice" or "too polite" or, frankly, too intimidated, we allowed the imposing party to dictate the terms of the interaction. We allowed ourselves to be nudged, ever so slightly, again and again and again, until we found ourselves stuck off-course in a conversational morass.

These interactions and impositions can have a cumulative effect. We can start to avoid places and activities we enjoy. We go to the other coffee shop around the corner because we don't want to see that one barista at our usual spot. We start hating work because we can't escape the complaining coworker. We stop going to the gym because Bob on the treadmill won't stop telling us about his gallstones. Or worse, we find ourselves becoming the imposers on the other end: has your significant other expressed frustration that all you do when you come home from work is bitch about Jerry, the jackass in the next cube? Has this started to have a negative impact on your relationship?

So the advice I want to share in this post is the following: When it comes to existing in the world, interacting with other members of the human species, dry land is a myth. We are all treading water: emotionally, financially, socially, romantically. It is my job to keep myself afloat, just as it is your job to keep yourself afloat. It is not my job to buoy you, nor is it your job to buoy me. If this sounds cruel, then it is useful to remember the advice given to those training in water rescue: if you approach a drowning person from the front it is common for them, in their desperation, to cling to you, and thus impede your ability to swim, and drown you both. The point is not that you should be indifferent to those who are failing to tread water; the point is that you are not helping them when you allow them to cling to you. You are only making the situation worse—and sometimes dire—for yourself.

There is a much broader issue at work here, and probably another blog post (pertaining to Americanized Judeo-Christian ideas about self-sacrifice and the deification of suffering, victim mentality, and inescapable individuality, etc.), but for the sake of this post the point is this: You have the right to decide how much of other people's garbage you want to carry. If someone tries to put their garbage in your lap, you are not a jerk for refusing it. They are the ones who are out of line. You don't have to be rude, you don't have to be cruel, you don't have to insult them or aggressively draw the line. But you do have the right to simply disengage.

Maybe one day we will all evolve and reach dry land, but until then just worry about keeping yourself afloat. I will, too.

IF YOU OWNED THE WHOLE WORLD, WHERE WOULD YOU KEEP IT?

Originally published on SuperheroSimplified.blogspot.com
July 15, 2014

If you owned the whole world, where would you keep it?

It's a serious question, so think about it for a second. Where would you put all of those cars and houses? Where would you put all of those iPads and football stadiums and Vera Wang shoes? You would have to put them someplace.

And where would you put the rivers and the forests? Where would you put the islands and the mountains? Where would you put the continents and the oceans? What cosmic door would you lock them behind to let others know that the world and its contents are yours and no one else's?

We spend a great deal of time in this life asking the important questions: What type of breakfast cereal do I like? What's my favorite flavor of cupcake? What kind of car do I want to drive? What unique seasonal Starbucks coffee beverage satisfies my personal palate? What kind of paddle board yoga fits my unique personhood? What color tank top looks best on me? What sunglasses should I wear? What team do I want to win? What bands and TV shows and movies do I like? What political view do I espouse? What style of decor do I prefer?

We are social primates, and as such we orient ourselves in reality by orienting ourselves within our group. We use such delineations ("My friends and I get together to binge watch *Orange is the New Black*"; "My friends and I watch the game every Sunday"; "My friend and I had bad service at ____ and swore we would never go back there," etc.) to assuage our fear of isolation (being left out of the group) and lack (fear that we will be denied access to the group because we fundamentally lack some resource—or the means to acquire some resource—which others possess or possess the means to acquire). Accordingly, the material artifacts of our own existence hold magical powers (they make us "belong"; they earn us regard within our social group's hierarchy) and operate within a rarified realm of superstition and irrationality: "I don't want to get rid of that ____," we think, remembering 1) good times we had with our group in the company of, or as a result of, ____, and 2) envisioning a potential future in which such good times might again occur, and 3) recoiling from the prospect of a time when, faced with the possibility of such future good times (togetherness! belonging!), we are denied those good times because we got rid of ____. Or we pine after something we do not yet possess, imagining a potential future in which possessing the coveted object will, like a magical talisman, produce an occurrence in which we experience profound validation and belonging...

I am not talking about true material lack, but rather perceived material lack: the desperate sense that I live on the brink of expulsion, that I am one bad outfit or wrong opinion away from crippling alienation. It's little wonder: we are bombarded almost constantly by the implied message (threat?) that somewhere some people in a social group (a social group to which we would like to belong) are having an amazing time, the kind of amazing time we always wanted to have but might never ever have, and all we need to do to join them is buy this brand of beer or this kind of car. We are told in a thousand subtle (and not-so-subtle) ways on a daily basis that this brand of soap or this kind of breakfast cereal will palliate our soul-deep fear that we will one day be left helpless and alone. (Seem like an exaggeration? Grocery shopper mom sees the commercial in which the good commercial mom gives her kids _____ for breakfast; the kids go off to school happy and ready to succeed; the bus driver or teacher notices the great conditions of the kids, and gives commercial mom an approving nod; commercial mom's efforts are validated, her value as a person within a community is reaffirmed; shopper mom throws the cereal in the cart, feeling good about what she's doing, even if she's not exactly sure why she's doing it...)

We are initiated into a narrative in which we, the protagonist, must seek the magical elixir to balm the unresolved ache at the core of our being (the ache of being inherently alienated, autonomous; the fear of this alienation). And yet it is the elixir itself which contains this narrative: "You know how you feel bad sometimes, even though you're not sure why?" it says. "The reason you feel bad is that you didn't have me!"

Thus we are told a story of want, of lack, of yearning: we are led down corridors of thought until we arrive at the door of fear (that I won't have what I need at the moment I need it; that this will alienate me from the group; that the group's derision will turn on me). We are told this story a hundred (a thousand?) times day. We ponder it when we are at the store, we hear it in advertisements, etc. Soon we have spent our whole lives meditating on need and lack: no sooner have we assuaged the yearning prompted by one false elixir than another clues us in to that elixir's failure. "You're still not happy!" it says. "But if you only owned me..."

Of course, the vast majority of us lack for nothing of any importance. We never miss a meal. We never sleep out in the elements. We never go without shoes or warm-enough clothes. In fact, given this low standard for what could be called "comfortable," many of us exist in a state of staggering opulence, surrounded by far more than we need. And yet so many of us live our lives consumed by thoughts of what we don't have, by fear of a potential future in which we will experience lack. Thus we accumulate, we hold onto, we store away, we stockpile, we do not share: we lock things behind doors and declare that they are ours and no one else's, never quite assuaging our needling anxiety that one day all will be lost (to disaster or disease or robbery or whatever else), that we need to stockpile more, to more vigilantly safeguard the castle walls of our own physical cache...

Let me put your mind at ease. One day you definitely will lose everything. One day, without a doubt, all of your stuff will stop being your stuff. All of the good times will end, and other people (people you want to be friends with!) will have fantastic good times without you. It's pretty much the single guarantee in life: that one day the whole thing is going to move on without you.

So let me offer you an alternative view. If you were able to constantly placate this anxiety, to acquire endlessly, until you owned the whole world, where would you keep it? You can answer the question however you want, but as far as I can see the thing that makes the most sense is to keep it right where it is. Everything already has a place.

So how would it then be yours, you ask? How would you ensure unfettered access to it? Perhaps an agreement would be made, between you and the citizens of the whole world, that whenever you showed up and needed ____, your ownership would be honored. In the mean time people could continue to live in your houses, sleep in your beds, eat your food, grow crops in your fields, and you, owner of all, would need to keep nothing separate, having access to all, always, everywhere.

Does this sound fantastic? It might, and yet this more accurately reflects the state of our lives: there is basically nothing that we could possibly want, in a given moment, that we could not soon acquire. Why, then, do we allow our fear of a potential future lack to dictate our behavior? Why, when history rather reflects perpetual access and abundance? Would it not be more reasonable to assume that, if I give away this table, there will be other tables in my future, should I require one?

There is a real danger that this essay will be dismissed as unforgivably "first world," as seemingly blind to the fact that in many parts of the world there is true lack and suffering. But it is rather exactly with this disparity in mind that I am writing this: If it is my own irrational and culturally encouraged fear of lack which causes me to lock my cupboard doors and say that everything inside is mine, regardless of all other need—even when my neighbor is starving—then it seems to me that by contemplating the true plenty of my life I will become more likely to unlock those doors and offer up what is inside.

So I encourage you to ask yourself: What do I need? If you cannot realistically imagine a scenario in which those needs are not met, then regard with suspicion the next advertisement that prompts your longing, that seems to promise an impossible state of transcendent happiness, a balm for your lack. Regard with considered suspicion the sense that, though you haven't worn that coat in ten years, you're not sure you want to give it away just yet. Be wary of material accumulation acting as a manifestation of fear.

YOU'RE NOT A KID ANYMORE

Originally published on SuperheroSimplified.blogspot.com
August 18, 2014

I made a new friend the other day. I'll call him Sarge. Sarge trains Brazilian Jiu-Jitsu at another school in the area, and he came and trained with us for a night. After class and open mat, as we were sitting around talking, Sarge said, "Realistically, I don't know how much longer I'm going to be doing this." He went on to list the (unfortunately, fairly typical) complaints that seem to plague most middle-aged American men. His knees hurt. His back hurts. He's not recovering the way he used to. Bumps and bruises, twists and sprains, don't disappear overnight anymore.

Sarge is a blue belt (for those of you who don't do BJJ: blue is the first belt after white, and comes before purple, brown, and finally black). He's "young" in Jiu-Jitsu years—it's common to spend 2 or more years at each belt level, and they say it takes on average 10 years to get a black belt—but he's already thinking about the day when he's going to hang up his gi: not because he wants to, but because he feels that, physically, he'll have to.

If you've been reading this blog for any length of time, you already know that I think Brazilian Jiu-Jitsu is an amazing art. Its efficacy as a fighting style is only the beginning. Many (if not most) other martial arts being taught today pay a lot of lip service to concepts like personal growth and character development, but their training practices and advancement policies have been softened to accommodate a larger clientele base, and their "challenges" have been so defanged that now the rank of black belt is accessible to children.

Don't get me wrong. I think that all martial arts have value: often in terms of the technical elements that they teach (to varying degrees), but always in terms of the benefit they can offer their students. However, the self-refinement that BJJ demands—the exposure of and rumination on personal (physical, technical, and most often mental and emotional) weakness—has the potential to produce a profound—and profoundly positive—change that can permeate and benefit all aspects of a practitioner's life. The physical aspect—what happens on the mat—is, as Bruce Lee's character said in *Enter the Dragon*, just the "finger pointing toward the moon."

Which is why it bothered me so much, when Sarge said what he said. Here was this guy—just a baby by Jiu-Jitsu standards—with so much benefit ahead of him, thinking he was probably going to have to quit, thinking he wasn't going to be up for the physical aspect—the finger pointing toward the moon—anymore.

There is a bit of a cultural rift happening in Jiu-Jitsu these days. Ryron and Rener Gracie, grandsons of the art's founder Helio Gracie and head instructors at the Gracie Jiu-Jitsu Academy in California, are encouraging students to "keep it playful" on the mats: to treat training as a game, not a competition. The vocal opposition takes the stance that Jiu-Jitsu is about fighting, and a fight is never a game: that the "keep it playful" mentality weakens Jiu-Jitsu. Proponents of this view encourage practitioners to treat training more like competition, and to regard injury, soreness, etc., as simply the cost of doing business.

If you train with me, you know where my opinion falls on this spectrum. However, I would be loathe to assert that one of these approaches is "right." Different people come to Jiu-Jitsu looking for different things, and I sincerely believe that everyone, no matter their approach, mindset, etc., walks off the mat benefitted in some way. I will say, however, that I don't enjoy training when every match is a death match. Moreover, for myself, I don't see the benefit that justifies the cost (i.e. injury, exhaustion, etc.). I don't see what is gained from this approach that isn't more effectively gained in other ways. Further, I think this approach fundamentally encourages attribute-based Jiu-Jitsu (moves and techniques that work because of specific size, strength, and conditioning elements related to the conditions present on a given day on a given time against a specific opponent) and, in rewarding it (the "what" of the victory is more important than the "how" of the victory) dis-incentivizes the search for fundamental principles that transcend the specifics of time and conditioning and opponent.

I write this knowing that these statements might easily be used to justify laziness, or to passive-aggressively disparage the victories of those of greater physical prowess. If you've read this blog or if you train with me then you already know how heavily I prioritize physical fitness. I consider myself and my students representatives of an art form and a tradition that carry a high standard, and I expect all of us to meet that standard. But I also know that my physical attributes, as much as I would like them to, aren't going to stick around forever. What's that old saying? Father Time is undefeated? One day that spring is going to be gone from my step. One day I'm not going to be able to out-scramble the hard-charging blue belts. And when that day comes, I want to know the core techniques that will work regardless. I want to know how to manage someone with position and leverage, not just grit and determination.

Which brings me back to Sarge. To hear Sarge tell it, Father Time is creeping up on him. To say that it sucks is a waste of breath. It's bigger than judgement. It's just inevitable. Our opinion has nothing to do with it. All we can do, really, is manage the process, and training Jiu-Jitsu like you're twenty-one—and thinking that you have to quit because you can't compete attribute-to-attribute against twenty-one-year-olds—is wrong. It's a waste. It's throwing the baby out with the bathwater.

So here's my advice to Sarge, and my advice to all of you: the pajama wrestling that we call Brazilian Jiu-Jitsu is only the tip of the iceberg. Don't make the mistake of thinking that the only thing of value to be gleaned from training is "victory" on the mat. Don't get locked into one concept of what Jiu-Jitsu looks like. Yes, it looks like a twenty-one-year-old physical specimen tearing up the mats and choking the daylights out of people. But it also looks like Helio Gracie, at 80 years old, defending, playing, and escaping against world champions less than half his age (that's not hyperbole: Saulo Ribeiro talks about it in his book). I truly believe that Jiu-Jitsu is for everyone. But, it's like that thing Einstein said: "Everybody is a genius. But if you judge a fish by its ability to climb a tree, it will live its whole life believing that it is stupid." If you judge yourself, at 45, by your ability to possess or employ the attributes of someone half your age, you will leave the mats feeling like Jiu-Jitsu isn't for you. And that, more than any victory or defeat on the mats, is the real loss.

FEAR IS A LIAR

Originally published on SuperheroSimplified.blogspot.com
October 6, 2014

It's getting to be Halloween season, so what better subject for a blog post than fear?

The human brain is an incredible thing, but it does have one or two little quirks. Chief amongst these is its over-developed (in comparison to other animals') ability to conceive of potential threats. You show me a playground and I'll show you a nervous mother who, with little to no prep time, could tell you a hundred ways her child could be horribly maimed or worse by any otherwise seemingly innocuous facet of the apparatus. "A child could fall off the swing," she might say. Or: "Those metal bolt-ends will rust sooner or later, and then it's tetanus central!"

Of course, this ability has served us well. We, the naked apes, have somehow managed to endure in some of the harshest climates and under some of the harshest circumstances we can imagine. And, for as much as we like to pat ourselves on the back and talk about the indomitable human spirit and the strength of grit and determination, our survival has been largely due not to our toughness but to this particular brand of cleverness: we know the winter is coming, so we harvest in the fall; we know the slide has rusty edges, and so we don't let our children play on it.

In short: we can see what might happen before it happens, and thus we are able to avoid myriad dangers both likely and unlikely.

But therein lies the (potential) problem. We are able to conceive of potentially disastrous outcomes, but somewhat less well-equipped when it comes to weighing (and dismissing) those outcomes. Simply put, we do not know what is going to happen, but we do know that we cannot predict the future, and likewise know too that we are unable to rule out any potential future (unable to say, with absolute authority, that this or that thing "cannot happen"). In short, we doubt our ability to make any assertion about the future, and in this doubt myriad and fearful potentialities may flourish, potentialities which we lack the authority to dismiss.

Please note: I am not saying that we are all irredeemably terrible at dismissing some of the more ludicrous possibilities. I am saying that we are not as good at dismissing them as we are at coming up with them. Once we come up with one, it is far too easy for doubt to linger.

Of course, experience is the great predictor: having walked down a path once, I am much more confident in my theory of what the experience will be the next time (a theory that replicates my previous experience). A walk down a street in a "bad" neighborhood is less fearful when we are bolstered by the knowledge that we have already passed this way once, and experienced no disaster. Any potentially dangerous act (and isn't every act "potentially dangerous"?), repeated often enough, loses its immediate fearfulness and takes on the quality of the mundane, the everyday.

But is this the only way to overcome fear? To do the fearful thing until it no longer frightens us? To dismiss the vision of the potential disaster only by bludgeoning and blunting it against experience?

If there is another way forward, it hinges on looking at fear itself, and explicating its premise and its implied reward.

Fear is not the event itself: fear lives in the anticipation of the event. In this way it is a form of time travel: we imagine a potential future *and* we experience an emotional response in the present (the potential future becomes physically real). More than this, we imagine a future self: a "me" that is living the experience I want to avoid (even when I am not aware of it, this potential me is always an implied part of any imagined future: I am always projecting about my own experience). When we imagine this person, this potential me, we step out of our present experience and experience instead a potential future (or series of potential futures) and, with it, experience the physical symptoms of the non-reality: we become nervous, our heart races, we may become defensive, or shy, or upset, or present any number of fear's symptoms. And yet here it is: the same safe present, the same beautiful day...

For what reason are we willing to tolerate fear intruding on the present in this fashion? For what fear offers in return: the fantasy of a future without calamity. "Pay attention to me," fear says, "and I will carry you safely through this world forever. You will never experience hardship or pain. I will protect you." Lulled by this promise we forgo the present and live always thirty seconds (or sixty minutes, or three days, or twenty years) in the future, mining the path ahead for potential threats while the world (our very lives) pass around us, unseen.

And yet: what is the appeal of this promise? That one day we will have negotiated all threats, illuminated all potential dangers, and then we will be free to forgo fear? Impossible: to live in the world is to have a physical body, is to attach to others and love them; in this there is no permanent safety. Perhaps the promise, then, is that no disaster will ever befall us! Again, impossible: a life lived in fear and a life lived without fear each end regardless; there is no escaping the final calamity. The promise, then, is that we will be free from suffering until that final calamity comes! Equally impossible: disaster may always come, unanticipated and unheralded, and to live in perpetual fear (inventing potential disaster after potential disaster, so that they may be avoided) is to live in perpetual horror of the future, to suffer inside the prison of fear.

Fear offers nothing that it can actually deliver. Fear is a liar. The only solution, then, is to regard fear as one regards an untrustworthy acquaintance: one that truly believes that, despite his many previous failures, this time he really will do what he promises. He will ardently plead with you, he will make a convincing case, and he will promise you a better future if you only just listen to him and do what he is asking. But of course, you know better by now. And so you refuse to live 30 seconds (or sixty minutes, or three days, or twenty years) in the future.

What remains? The eternal present, the only true reality you know, ever knew, will ever know (despite fear's promises and warnings). And the knowledge that disaster may come at any moment, anticipated or not: that fear does not mitigate the potentialities it describes (nor does it often predict the true horrors we face), and the gratitude when the present moment is pleasant, is not one eaten up with the thousand natural shocks that flesh is heir to.

THE PAST IS OVER

Originally published on SuperheroSimplified.blogspot.com
January 1, 2015

"In our day, when historical pressure no longer allows any escape, how can man tolerate the catastrophes and horrors of history— from collective deportations and massacres to atomic bombings—if beyond them he can glimpse no sign, no transhistorical meaning; if they are only the blind play of economic, social, or political forces, or, even worse, only the result of the 'liberties' that a minority takes and exercises directly on the stage of universal history?... We know how, in the past, humanity has been able to endure the sufferings we have enumerated: they were regarded as a punishment inflicted by God, the syndrome of the decline of the 'age,' and so on. And it was possible to accept them precisely because they had a metahistorical meaning... Every war rehearsed the struggle between good and evil, every fresh social injustice was identified with the sufferings of the Saviour (or, for example, in the pre-Christian world, with the passion of a divine messenger or vegetation god), each new massacre repeated the glorious end of the martyrs... By virtue of this view, tens of millions of men were able, for century after century, to endure great historical pressures without despairing, without com-

mitting suicide or falling into that spiritual aridity that always brings with it a relativistic or nihilistic view of history."
—Mircea Eliade, *The Myth of the Eternal Return*

There's a storyline in one issue of *Savage Sword of Conan* (don't ask me which, I read it fifteen years ago, and Google isn't getting me anywhere) in which Conan, sworn to help the endangered people of some proto-African tribe, but grievously ill (or wounded, or both, I can't remember), is possessed by the spirit of the tribe's patron defender, by virtue of an endlessly-repeated magical incantation voiced by the village's Shaman/Medicine Man/Priest, and is able to carry out his mission, i.e. kill an entire tribe's worth of attacking warriors, until the Shaman/Medicine Man/Priest stops repeating the magical incantation, and Conan collapses, insensate, with no memory of what happened.

So what does this have to do with the new year, the phenomenon of transhistorical meaning, and the myth of the eternal return?

The past is a funny thing. We take it for granted that past events are real, irreducible: that they retain their permanent reality, even when no physical trace of them remains. We shudder at the thought that anything might be forgotten, negated by the passage of time: we erect monuments to the fallen so that their brave actions "will not have been in vain," i.e. allowed to disappear into the nothingness of all that has been forgotten.

Indeed, there seems little so viscerally terrifying as this negation: the thought that our actions come, finally, to nothing; that all we love and hold most precious will disappear entirely, never to reappear. I remember laying awake as a child, grappling with the suffocating thought that one day I would die, and that then I would be dead forever.

Thoughts like these are a short slip down a slippery slope to abject nihilism. Why do anything? One day you'll be dead and then you'll be forgotten, and then all of your earthly efforts will receive history's final, amnesiac valuation.

It is healthier, finally, to ignore this looming truth. It's hard to function otherwise. So we compose our thoughts in such a way that our actions seem to matter, have substance: I do A which allows me to do B; B allows C, C allows D... Each thing gives purpose to the one preceding, in a chain whose final terminus I don't consider.

Yet this wholly forgivable and arguably necessary existential apparatus can quickly become a trap: the permanent past is carved in stone, inalterable, for good or ill. Accordingly, the self crystalizes, petrifies: I will always be the person who did A, we think; I will always be the person who didn't do B; I will always be the person to whom C occurred. We see the behaviors of the past as manifestations of an essential self, an irreducible ME: we feel beholden to them, culpable for them, a permanent fixed present referent for all of our past sins and transgressions.

And yet what reality do these past occurrences have? The majority leave no trace, and the physical marks (scars, damage, etc.) that do remain must glean their meaning anew each day (each moment) from the repeated incantation of their origin and meaning. "That's the field where it happened," we think as we look at the expanse, while to another viewer, uninitiated into our private world of meaning, the field means nothing at all. The field is the field, only: its specific contours send no shiver of sorrow or joy through the mind of the uninformed. And yet the reality we consider seems as permanent, as irrefutable, as immitigable as if it is occurring again, as if it never stopped occurring...

In his book *The Myth of the Eternal Return* (which I quoted at the beginning of this post), novelist and philosopher Mircea Eliade makes the case that the perception of the *de facto* truth of linear time (as opposed to circular time) is a modern invention, a modern presumption: that the sense of history as ever-accumulating is a modern contrivance, no more essentially true (since the past lives primarily as an epistemological construction of the present) than the contrary notion that linear time's events are insubstantial, and that only the essential cycle (annual death and rebirth) holds preeminent and transcendent value. I mention it here (and at the beginning of the post) not to argue the merits of this philosophy in an essential way, but in a personal way: imagine yourself not as the accumulation of your past, but rather as a being made of your own unconscious and constant recitation of that past, a construction which, like Conan possessed by the defender spirit, will collapse without this constant reiteration of its own existence: a being which may be born anew at each moment simply by that being altering the nature of its own self-incantation.

In short: 1) that the past holds preeminent existential value as a method for self-construction and self-definition, 2) that the past, having no present reality, is essentially only the story told about the past, and is as such as insubstantial as any other story, having only the value and weight ascribed it by the speaker and listener(s) and 3) that the story may be thus modified, altered, revised, or forgotten entirely.

Am I suggesting, then, that we pass ourselves off as what we are not, to impress chicks and get free drinks? Certainly not. Being free from the past does not make you anything more than free from the past. Becoming something else is the work of the present. I am suggesting, however, that you not allow your past to become or remain the prison of your present. In this new year, remember that you have the freedom and the power and the authority to make yourself anew.

Wishing you all a safe and happy and most of all, SUPER new year.

WHAT I'VE BEEN THINKING LATELY REGARDING BELT RANK IN BJJ

Originally Posted on Facebook on August 19, 2013
Published on SuperheroSimplified.blogspot.com
January 22, 2015

For anyone interested, this is what I've been thinking about lately regarding belt rank.

I got my brown belt from Steve Maxwell in the spring of 2012, and since then I've spent a lot of time (a lot more time than I did at any previous rank, including in other martial arts) thinking about rank and what it means.

Part of this has to do with really, really wanting the black belt. Pretty much from the moment the brown belt went around my waist I started thinking about the next time my belt would change. I started asking myself the questions that brown belts ask themselves: What do I have to do to get my black belt? What's the difference between me now and the me I need to be? What will it mean when my belt changes? What internal alteration will that symbolize?

When you start Brazilian Jiu-Jitsu, the black belt seems impossibly far away. You hear stories about Caio Terra and BJ Penn getting their black belts in record time, but you also hear horror stories about guys condemned to one lower rank or another for three or four or five years. You hear the commonly-repeated estimate that it takes about ten years for the typical student to earn his or her black belt. Coming up in Northeast Ohio in the mid-aughts, the mystique of the black belt was compounded by the fact that you never met any: black belts were few and far between. Like many people, my first instructor wasn't a black belt: he was a *blue belt* at the time. "Geez," I used to think, "If I have to be as good as Darren to get even a blue belt, I'll never be good enough to be a black belt."

There's another maxim that gets thrown around: A black belt is just a white belt who never gave up. Sooner or later we all climbed the ranks, and guys I knew started getting blues and purples and browns. Then, suddenly, somebody had their black belt. Then somebody else. And even though those guys were good, they didn't fly or walk on water. They were still the same guys, still good at some stuff and needing work on other stuff, still susceptible to the guillotine or late on the sprawl, or whatever.

They were still just students, just like me, just trying to get better.

Anything so coveted is bound to breed strong feelings, and often times those feelings are ones of jealousy and resentment. These feelings are often fueled by the discrepancy we find between our perception of what a black belt should be (a superhero!) and the guys we see with the belt around their waists. "He only got the belt because _____," we say, for some reason oblivious to the fact that, once this conversation starts, it will sooner or later come back around to shine its harsh light on us, and our rank...

About the worst thing you can say about someone in BJJ is that he's over-ranked. Say he's over-ranked and you dismiss him outright, while simultaneously calling into doubt the credibility of his school and his instructor and his association. It's like calling someone a "thief" or a "coward" in the Old West: it's a stain, a mark that's easy to apply and hard to wash off. I've heard this term used to describe black belts and I've heard it used to describe four-stripe white belts. What's more: I've used it. I used it as a tough, strong, athletic white belt to describe blue and purple belts that I made "really work to tap me." I used it as a strong, smashy blue belt to describe purple belts that I "almost tapped."

In other words: I used it to bolster my ego at someone else's expense, when I envied their rank or when I didn't like that they'd tapped me, or when I felt lousy for one of any of a hundred other reasons. I used it the same way any schoolyard bully calls someone else a cruel name to allay his own feelings of self-doubt and fear.

(And, just as an aside: The flip side of this coin is saying that a guy is under-ranked. This can be done in a complimentary fashion: "You feel great, bro. You definitely feel like a ____ belt!" But here, too, we sometimes find the fear lurking: "I can't believe a ____ belt gave me so much trouble; that guy is under-ranked! He should be a ____ belt!" We protect ourselves, forgive ourselves for our failings by elevating the status of the force against which we failed.)

What horrible-seeming truth was I hiding from? That I wasn't as good as I thought I was, when I imagined myself rolling? That I wasn't the second coming of Rickson? That I didn't actually deserve my blue or my purple or my whatever belt, like I (in my expert opinion) felt I did? Fear that the tenuous strands of success I had lashed together to form an image of myself about which I could feel pride would crumble and fall at the first suggestion that I still had room to improve, to grow? That I wasn't perfect yet?

No one—Helio Gracie included—ever said that strength and toughness *weren't* a consideration in a fight. In fact, Gracie Jiu-Jitsu could be said to be founded on the exact opposite idea: that a strong guy is always going to be dangerous, and a smaller, weaker man needs technique and strategy to not only survive this danger, but *prevail*. I think many of us labour under the delusion (and it's an old delusion, a carry-over from the heyday of Karate in the '80s) that once we master this art and these skills all altercations will be effortless: that we will be so far above any attack anyone could mount that our assailants will simply fly off of us like bullets off Superman's chest. But this is, and always was, a fairy tale: a strong guy is a strong guy is a strong guy; a tough guy is a tough guy is a tough guy. Jiu-Jitsu is there so that these advantages may be managed and overcome: not dismissed or negated outright.

Strength and toughness have no belt rank. They don't even have any obvious characteristics. I outweigh the strongest guy I've ever rolled with by probably twenty pounds. You would never think to look at him that he's as freakishly strong as he is. What are you going to do? Some guys are strong. Some guys are tough. Rolling with this guy is work. Does it matter that his belt is white? Some, certainly. But definitely not as much as you'd like it to.

And, as a related note, if you didn't know this already, let me tell you now: brown belts (or at least the one's I've talked to about this) hate rolling with white and blue belts. (Note # 1: This isn't everybody. I've rolled with a lot of nice white and blue belts. Note # 2, to my students: I'm not talking about you.) I'm talking about walking into another school and feeling the white and blue belts look at you and think: here's a chance to put a notch in my belt. If I can tap the brown belt, if I can make the brown belt work to tap me, I must be good. I must be tough, I must be X, Y, Z. They look at you as a way to build themselves up by putting you down, and it is a toxic energy that you can physically feel when rolling with them.

Wearing a white belt doesn't make you a wimpy weakling, anymore than wearing a brown belt makes me a superhero. I feel like this is something a lot of us, at lower ranks, lose sight of. Inside of that gi is a person. He's made of the same stuff as you. He breaks like you break. Just because he's wearing a brown belt it does not mean that you're allowed to go at him with reckless indifference to his health and wellbeing.

If I have a brown belt around my waist, it doesn't mean I'm a brown belt at everything I do. I have stuff I just learned last week, just like you. I have my white belt stuff, and I have my blue belt stuff, and I may even have some black belt stuff. But I don't need to work on my brown and black belt stuff as much as I need to work on my white and blue belt stuff. And if you're going to come at me like you want to kill me, like they're going to crown you king of the mat if you tap me, then I can't roll with you with my white belt stuff. I can't play. I can't experiment. I can't work on what I need to work on to grow. And that means you are wasting my time and energy. And that's not ok.

So we're back to the question: What does rank mean? What are the belts there for, if white belts can be tough and brown belts can be weak? What does my brown belt mean, if I still have white belt parts of my game? What does any belt objectively mean?

I'm a big believer in Malcolm Gladwell's 10,000 hour theory of mastery, described in his book *Outliers*. For anyone who hasn't read it (or his other books *Blink*, *The Tipping Point*, and *What the Dog Saw*) I recommend you start as soon as you're finished with this. The 10,000 hour theory basically states that it takes 10,000 hours to master any body of knowledge. Talent helps, intelligence helps, but the most important thing is putting in the time. Basically the idea is that there are certain insights you only come to once you have considered a body of knowledge for a given period: at 3,000 hours you understand the subject one way; at 5,000 you understand it another way; at 7,000 your understanding has once again changed; at 10,000 you've looked at it from more angles than almost anyone else, and your insights and conclusions are a product of this extensive experience.

Imagine a ladder 10,000 rungs high. Imagine the 10,000th rung as the great insight, the stroke of genius. Nobody—not Steve Jobs or Bill Gates or Einstein—got to that 10,000th rung by jumping from the 3,000th, or the 5,000th, or the 8,000th. They got to that rung from the one below it, and to that one from the one below that, and to that one from the one below that...

Now let's imagine you go into a woodworking shop, and you're going to build a cabinet. And the master woodworker is there, and you're each going to build a cabinet. You start talking about how you're going to go about it. The master woodworker describes the methods he's going to use, and the details he's going to incorporate, and on and on. To you, this is all gibberish: right now you're worried about putting together something that will work, basically, and his talk is just taking up your time. So you both build a cabinet, and hours later you've built a functional cabinet, and he's built a beautiful cabinet: but one that isn't any better at holding books or dishes or whatever than yours is.

Whose approach is better? Which cabinet is better?

The answer is: It doesn't matter. You both built a cabinet. The master woodworker's cabinet benefits from his 10,000 hours of experience, and is different from yours in a thousand ways, but these differences are largely only the master woodworker's concern. Moreover, the differences are a blur to you. You can't even begin to understand why he did things the way he did them, or how. Not because you're dumber, or less talented, or a worse woodworker, but because you're not looking at the two cabinets from the 10,000th rung. You're looking at them from the 1st rung, and the view is very different.

I didn't say worse. I said different.

So what is that belt around your waist supposed to tell you? It's supposed to tell you who your peers are. It's supposed to tell you: These people are also at the 3,000th, or 4,000th, or 8,000th rung. These people are looking at the same things you're looking at, thinking about the same things you're thinking about. These are the people who can best help you reach your next rung, and not necessarily by being your toughest opponents. Not necessarily by fighting you to the death. Not necessarily by pushing you to your physical limit. They're the ones who understand what you're doing, and can give you the most constructive feedback. That's it.

One of my favorite anecdotes about the old Gracie Academy is that there were only three belts: white, light blue, and dark blue. The belts weren't given according to skill. The dark blue belts were students who had completed the instructor course, and were certified to teach. The light blue belts were currently enrolled in the instructor course, but hadn't completed it yet. Everyone else wore a white belt.

This is my philosophy of rank: We are all white belts. A student of Gracie Jiu-Jitsu is a student of Gracie Jiu-Jitsu is a student of Gracie Jiu-Jitsu is a student of Gracie Jiu-Jitsu. We are all white belts. Nobody is "done." We're all getting on the mat to try to reach our next rung. If you tap a higher ranked student, good for you. If a lower ranked student taps you, good for him. But don't get too hung up on either. Neither really amounts to much. You're as good as you are. If someone taps you, you're still as good as you are. If you tap someone else, you're still as good as you are. You are where you are, and other people are where they are. You're on the rung you're on, and that's it.

Whatever color the belt around my waist is, I'll see you on the mats tonight. And even though I want the black belt, I know that all I'll have to say on the day it gets tied around my waist is: I'll see you on the mats tonight. And I'll be fumbling around like always, looking for the next rung.

RUSSIAN PENICILLIN

Originally published on SuperheroSimplified.blogspot.com
August 24, 2015

I hate going to the doctor. I know there are a lot of great doctors out there, but too many of the ones I've visited seem overconfident and under-productive. Nine times out of ten, the experience puts me in mind of Voltaire's observation that "[t]he art of medicine consists of keeping the patient amused while nature heals the disease." Which would be all well and good, were it not for the bill. I'm certainly not the first person to observe that the healthcare system has gone off the rails—that one shouldn't have to decide between treating an illness and making a car payment—but that is beyond the scope of this post. Today's post is about skipping the trip to the doctor entirely.

Before I go any further, I will say that—of course—there are innumerable ailments for which prompt medical treatment is advised. Considering both the financial and health impacts of the most common modern medical interventions (prescription medications—especially antibiotics—and surgery) I certainly wouldn't fault anyone a moment's hesitation. However, when in doubt, go see a doctor. I am not one.

And a note about health: the traditional germ theory of disease holds that illness is caused by the presence of germs. The individual comes in contact with an infecting bacteria or virus, and this bacteria or virus makes them ill. This theory, though widely held by the public (hence the ever-increasing popularity of Purell), is now being seen as incomplete by many doctors. The (actually, not so) new theory holds that illness is the product of a confluence of factors, involving the strength of the infecting organism and the weakness of the host. This revision begins to return focus to the human immune system as both the primary and the ideal respondent when a disease is present. Accordingly, any discussion of illness is really a discussion about overall health, as an illness indicates a weakening of the overall organism. Treatment must, therefore, include steps to identify and remove those stresses which so reduced the organism's energies in the first place that the disease was able to proliferate. For myself, I've found that my periods of un-wellness correspond almost exclusively with periods of marked overtraining. You may have noticed such correlations yourself, in periods where you don't get as much sleep as you should, or when work makes new and heightened demands, or when your diet isn't as good as it should be. Quick and effective recovery from any illness must begin with the identification and, if not outright elimination, mitigation of these stressors.

In previous posts, I've discussed various practices designed to make us healthier, i.e. more resistant to disease. Today I want to talk a bit about the other side of the coin—what to do when you're already afflicted—and how garlic (nicknamed "Russian Penicillin" during WWII, because the Russian government, out of penicillin, literally started using garlic in its place) can save you recovery time and a doctor's bill.

When fresh garlic is crushed (or cut, but crushed is better) it produces a powerfully antibiotic, anti-fungal, and anti-viral compound called *allicin*. The allicin is at its peak ten to fifteen minutes after the garlic is crushed, and starts to degrade quickly after. A quick search online will discover many ailments for which fresh, crushed garlic has proven itself effective, but I have personally used it to treat the following:

SINUS/NASAL CONGESTION (sinus infection)

Cut two discs of garlic off a peeled clove and place one in each nostril. Try to breathe through your nose for as long as you can (pretty soon your nostrils will become blocked with all the gunk pouring out of your face). Try to keep the garlic in for ten minutes. Doing this more than once a day can irritate the delicate lining of the nasal passages, but just once a day has helped me kick some nasty congestion in no time.

SORE THROAT (strep)

Put a peeled clove of garlic in your mouth and suck on it like a lozenge. While you're doing that, bite through the outer skin. Not enough to break the clove apart, just enough to start releasing the juices. I've done this for as long as an hour with one clove.

EARACHE (ear infection)

I had a million ear infections as a kid, and a few as an adult. This method has worked better than any of the antibiotic drops I ever used: Crush a clove of garlic into a tablespoon of coconut or olive oil. Allow it to sit for ten minutes, then apply the garlic oil inside the afflicted ear with a q-tip or dropper. You can also buy soft-gel garlic supplements, and squeeze the contents into the afflicted ear. Done once or twice a day, this technique has cleared up some really painful earaches for me. Note that, if you suspect that your eardrum is ruptured, you don't want to pour anything in your ear.

RINGWORM

Sooner or later, if you're a grappler, you're going to get ringworm. It's practically a right of passage. Most over-the-counter anti-fungal medication say they can take up to two weeks to work. The last time I had ringworm, I knocked the sucker out in one day. Cut a disc from a peeled clove of garlic and tape it over the ring. Leave it on overnight. Note that even though the ring may scab over and look like it's dead, you should keep applying a coat of crushed garlic "juice" for at least a week to avoid recurrence and spreading the blight. Also: Don't grapple if you've got it. Keep it covered. Wash your gis with bleach or white vinegar.

WARTS

Similar method to treating ringworm. Crush a piece of garlic the size of the wart and place it over the wart. Tape in place. You want to leave this on pretty much all the time. Even though garlic is strong medicine, this method may take a few weeks, so be patient. And be consistent. I had a wart that the dermatologist tried to burn off, which left me with 1) a nasty scar, 2) a nasty bill, and 3) an undiminished wart. The garlic method did the trick, though. Alternately, a cotton swab soaked in apple cider vinegar, applied using the same protocol, is also effective.

STAPH

New research has shown that even the dreaded MRSA responds to garlic. I didn't have MRSA, but I did have a very angry staph infection on my leg (which included redness, swelling, and swollen lymph nodes) that topical garlic knocked out. Crush a clove, give it a few minutes to produce some allicin, smear the juices on the site, and cover with a bandage. I went a little too hard at this and actually burned the skin around the infection (I crushed a clove and then held it on for about ten minutes with a hot water bottle), but the kinder, gentler approach should produce rapid effects with little discomfort.

BRONCHITIS

Kicking the last of this right now, which is why I'm writing this post. For the past three weeks I've been dealing with a lingering and worsening cough. Too much Judo, too much strength training, too much teaching, too much dairy, and too much running around caught up with me. Finally I coughed up a little bit of blood, and I decided it was time to get serious. Three days of garlic therapy and I'm seeing light at the end of the tunnel. I haven't been messing around: I've been eating 3-5 (small) cloves of garlic a day. I chew the cloves until they're mush, and then swallow them. I'm also mega-dosing on vitamin C, eating primarily fruits and cooked vegetables, and cutting way back on the training. I've also been using the protocols for sore throat and sinus congestion as needed.

Among other things, I love that garlic has the potential to save you from taking a course of antibiotics. The dangers of antibiotic-resistant bacteria aside, a successful course of antibiotics decimates your gut flora, further compromising your already taxed immune system. I've seen different opinions on the subject, but there is evidence that garlic actually helps produce a favorable environment for healthy bacteria, while knocking out the baddies.

Please note that some people are allergic to garlic, so use caution when trying any of these methods for the first time. Also note that topical garlic can burn your skin, so don't leave the crushed clove on too long. A swab of juices alone tends not to burn me, but you may be more sensitive. Also note that not all garlic is created equal: irradiated garlic will not produce the allicin, and is little more than a flavoring agent (irradiation is commonly used to control pests). It's easy to tell if your garlic is irradiated: if the center of your clove has a green, still-growing stalk your garlic is not irradiated; if your garlic has a hollow tube in the center where the stalk should be, your garlic is irradiated and inert. Also note that garlic can act as a blood thinner, so you may want to consult with a doctor if you are already on blood thinners, or are pregnant or nursing. Also note that garlic is a powerful diuretic, so don't be surprised if you see increased output. And finally, it's worth noting that according to Reiki practitioners raw garlic is toxic to the energetic body, disrupting cross-brain communication. You can either believe in that or not, but it's probably not a bad idea to consider raw garlic strong medicine to be used as-needed.

Final note: If you eat a lot of garlic, it's totally normal to start smelling like garlic. Don't worry; the smell goes away once you stop eating the garlic. And as far as I'm concerned, it's a small price to pay for the benefit.

Until next time, folks: stay super.

IGNORE ALIEN ORDERS

Originally published on SuperheroSimplified.blogspot.com
September 24, 2015

To an infant, the world is meaningless.

I don't mean that infants are nihilists. I mean that infants are un-informed. They don't understand the relationship between heat and fire, between firecrackers and loud noises. They don't know what a kitchen mixer is, or how central heating works. It's all just noise and shape and movement.

As you grow out of infancy, your perspective becomes informed: by experience, by parents, by teachers, by social and political leaders, by TV and advertising, by religion, by the other kids at school. Piece by piece, you learn about your environment. You learn that some things are good, and some things are bad. You learn that some things are desirable, and some things aren't. You learn that wanting certain things is morally right, and wanting other things is morally wrong. You learn that what you want defines you as a type of person.

Maybe you learn that happiness or prosperity or abundance must be earned (the American dream of working yourself up from noth-ing; the Santa Claus archetype of the patron rewarding good behav-ior; St. Peter considering your resume before you're allowed to enjoy

Heaven). Maybe you learn that you don't deserve love unless you look, behave, or speak in a certain way. Maybe you learn that intelligence is the most desirable thing a person can possess: that lacking intelligence relegates you to a lesser quality of life. Or maybe you learn the same thing about athleticism, or charm, or creativity, or whatever.

Many of these lessons fall into a category we might call culturally-conferred survival intelligence. A thousand years ago this category would have included skills like hunting and fishing, finding water, building a shelter. Since you're reading this on the screen of an electrical device or in a mass-produced paperback book, I think it's probably safe for me to assume that for you this category includes things like understanding the specific fire dangers that exist in a modern home, or the knowledge for how to safely operate a motor vehicle, or knowing which neighborhoods to avoid.

Regardless of context, culturally-conferred survival intelligence is information about our environment that directly contributes to our ability to successfully navigate that environment.

However, while there is an undeniable survival value in integrating oneself into a group, it cannot be said that the majority of the lessons we learn are related to our survival in any essential way. Most are rather designed to inform our understanding of our social and cultural landscape, and draw their authority not from their inherent wisdom (i.e. "Don't touch snakes that look like that one or you will die,") but from the claimed or asserted moral authority of some governing body: God and the church; teachers and educational institutions; political leaders and society as a whole. While it would be foolish to suggest that such information is wholly useless, I do think it is useful to remember that these lessons and the institutions propagating and backing them are secondary layers imposed onto your consciousness from outside, designed to some extent to help you succeed but also, in many ways, to integrate you seamlessly into a pre-existing system.

I don't mean to suggest that there is a vast conspiracy in the works, designed to produce compliant and complicit cogs for a vast machine which is itself designed to retain power and influence for those who already possess it (or at least I don't mean to suggest it in this post). I mean only to point out that all such thoughts belonging to external systems function not out of any intrinsic moral authority and not with any true survival imperative, but largely to integrate your (foreign) consciousness into the existing system of thought, behavior, valuation, etc.

And I make this point because I think a lot of us walk around feeling conflicted within ourselves, unable to reconcile our desires and impulses with our informed feelings about those desires. We say things like, "I would love to have a job where I could sit at home and watch movies all day. But you can't do that. I've got to be a responsible adult." Or, "It was such a beautiful day today, I would have loved to have been out on the river fishing. Instead, I had to work." It is not simply a matter of a conflict existing between the impulse and the circumstances, but a conflict existing within our own minds: one part of the mind wants to go do something else, and another jumps up to enforce a restriction which, more often than not, has its origin in an external source.

We have learned that if you don't want to work at a job you don't like—if you don't want to spend the fleeting hours of your singular life in an environment you can't stand with people you don't want to be with—you're lazy and irresponsible, you're unrealistic, you're immature and childish. We have learned that if you would rather spend the rest of your life as a fishing guide somewhere beautiful it means you lack ambition. We teach our children that if they don't want to sit still for hours at a time, listening to a lesson on something they don't care about, then there is something wrong with them, and they need to behave better, and perhaps need to be medicated, etc. We teach young boys that wrestling and roughhousing—something all young mammals do—is wrong and deserving of punishment and rebuke.

We tell ourselves we should work harder, strive for a culturally-defined model of success, and disparage ourselves when we fall short. We participate endlessly in scripts that other people wrote, living someone else's version of success or parental love or aspiration or ambition. We accept the programming and we participate in it, and life goes by, and then it's over.

Am I saying you should quit your job and fish all day? Certainly not. I am saying that it is useful to remember that so many of our negative views about ourselves and our impulses or desires exist within systems of thought that were imposed upon us when we were young, and have been reinforced throughout our lives. I am saying, simply, that it can be useful to become aware of your thoughts' origin. Did they come from yourself, or were they imposed? Were they imprinted on you at a young age? Do they exist to mesh you seamlessly into an existing system? And if so: Is that system something in which you want to participate? Are you participating willingly, purposefully, of your own volition, or are you subservient to it? And if you are subservient: Will you continue to be your own watchdog, your own warden, continuously thwarting your own attempts to secede? Living in accordance with the law for the sake of ease and peace in my own life doesn't mean that I agree with the law, or even assent to its moral authority. I may live in a way that acknowledges its civic or judicial authority, and I may appreciate its purpose (laws allow us to live in close proximity to each other, all striving after the same things, without the whole thing devolving into chaos), but this does not mean that I must see myself (or my own "illegal" impulses) through the lens of that law's self-claimed moral authority.

We love the word "freedom" in this country. We trot it out on every patriotic occasion. We pat ourselves on the back for our freedom of religion and freedom of the press and our freedom from illegal search and seizure. But I worry that we've missed the point: that our forefathers set down these laws not for themselves but as a gesture toward a larger project, a broader effort to maintain a free

148

space in American life for philosophical diversity and spiritual growth: a free space in which we might stand unencumbered by the architecture of thought that various systems impose. To have a space in which we might claim our own moral authority, and define our own system of valuation, and hold it in higher esteem than the one implanted by a social machine.

In the end, no system is beholden to you. No system will save you. The group whose number you imagine you have joined by your participation will not notice when you fall from its ranks. To remain loyal to the system, beholden to it, subject and subservient to it, is to give your life away.

Don't do it. This life is *your* life. Make it super.

CHANGE

Originally published on SuperheroSimplified.blogspot.com
June 16, 2016

Listen. Here's the truth. NOBODY wants you to change. Not your family, not your friends, not even you.

You may think you want to change. Your friends and your family may think they want you to change. The truth is, though, they don't. When it comes right down to it—when it comes to the nitty-gritty work of changing day-to-day habitual behavior and modes of interacting—nobody wants you to do it.

Why not? Because all change—even positive change—is disorienting and stressful. It makes the known world unfamiliar again. It means taking a long hard second look at things that you take for granted. In short, it's work, and given the choice we'd all rather not work. When it comes right down to it, we'd all rather keep living in the world we know and understand, the one that's familiar, even if that world kind of sucks.

But here's the thing. You know you need to change. Part of you isn't satisfied. Part of you expects more of you. And when you walked into the gym for the first time, it was that part of you that was in the driver's seat.

Getting back in shape is hard. Getting better at BJJ is really hard. Confronting your own excuses and refusing to let them define you anymore is really, really hard. At some point along the way, it's normal for the part of you that expects more to get tired. And at that point it's normal to get frustrated, to feel like no one is giving you credit for the work you've done, for you to wish that someone would just tell you that what you've done is good enough already.

Here's the promise that I made to you when you walked in and became my student. Of all of the voices in your life that will tell you that you've tried hard enough, that you've done enough, that you're good enough, *I won't be one of them*. My job is to keep expecting more of you so that you keep expecting more of yourself. Not because you suck, or because you're a bad person, or because you're a loser, but because you are attempting something difficult and laudable, and it is my job as your coach and your instructor to facilitate and encourage that in every way that I can. It is my job to be the voice that says, "Keep pushing. Keep working. Keep expecting more."

So don't get discouraged. You're doing a good job. Now, do more of it.

CAGE-FREE
THOUGHTS ON THE FIGHT GYM'S — AND MY OWN — TRANSITION OUT OF MMA

Originally published on JiuJitsuDoMaeda.com
May 22, 2017

"The Stone Age did not end for lack of stone."
—Sheikh Ahmed Zaki Yamani

I often joke that, for whatever reason, I always just took it for granted that life meant getting punched in the face.

Blame Batman, maybe. Or, more likely, blame Steven Spielberg and the creative team behind the Indiana Jones movies. Here's ten-year-old Scott, transfixed in front of the TV, learning that, if you want to get anywhere in life, you're probably going to have to take a few cracks on the jaw.

It's not a bad lesson to learn, really, at least in the metaphorical sense. Fight for what you want, fight for what you believe in, get up when you get knocked down. Sure, it's a great lesson as a metaphor. But after almost twenty years in the martial arts, I feel qualified to tell you that it's not much of a fight strategy.

One of the first things they teach you in Gracie Jiu-Jitsu is that the most dangerous place to stand in a fight is at arm's length from your opponent. Farther away and he can't touch you, closer in and he's too jammed up to have much power. At arm's length, though, you're right there in his kill zone. The problem with the striking arts, the Gracies teach, is that in order for me to deploy my weapons—my strikes—I have to stand in what is, essentially, the most dangerous place to stand. Which I'll grant you is less of a concern when I'm the bigger, stronger, more durable fighter, but what about when I'm not? And, when it comes right down to it, why would I assume that I'm going to be? Who's going to pick a fight with me anyway, if not somebody bigger, stronger, and scarier?

Of course, smaller people do knock out bigger people. But bigger people knock out smaller people too, and considering the forces at play that's the far more likely outcome. And in a street fight situation, where your potentially unconscious head and body don't necessarily have a soft place to land, and where there's no guarantee of anyone stepping in to stop the punishment, a knockout can be a life-changing—if not life-ending—trauma. It's a big risk to take, and an awfully big risk to build into your fight strategy.

The notion that striking is actually an inferior strategy to grappling presents a challenging and potentially vertigo-inducing paradigm shift for those of us for whom "fighting" and "martial arts" and "self-defense" mean Bruce Lee and Jackie Chan, to say nothing of those of us with years already invested in the striking arts, and is met with resistance to this day. And, ironically enough, modern MMA in general and the UFC in particular are now held up as unassailable proof that Gracie Jiu-Jitsu is not enough, that striking arts are equally valid, that the time we've spent training Muay Thai or Boxing or Tae Kwan Do has not been wasted. The modern MMA fighter has to be good at everything to be successful, we all say, and accordingly modern MMA must be the ultimate martial art.

Back in 2006, that's how we thought of it, too. Back then, we saw Gracie Jiu-Jitsu as part of a broader skillset, something you had to train along with other arts in order to be "well-rounded." And so we trained in Muay Thai and Western Boxing and BJJ and American Wrestling, laboring under the notion that if we "filled the toolbox with tools"—if we got good enough at everything—then we could handle anything.

But go down this road even a little way, and you find that it's not really so simple: that, in fact, the situation becomes more problematic the more tools you have. A skill in the abstract is one thing, but the transition between abstract and application raises more essential questions. If six martial arts teach six different answers to a given situation, which one do you choose? Your opponent throws a jab: do you parry and counter like a boxer, or slip and shoot the double leg like a wrestler? Do you block his punch and work inside to establish your Muay Thai clinch? Of course, throughout a sparring match you will have multiple opportunities to try out each of these options, but what if this isn't a friendly sparring match? What if there are no gloves and no round timers, just someone big enough and strong enough that their jab is liable to break your jaw? Are you 100% confident that you'll pick the right approach when the first punches are already flying at your head? When a knockout can mean a trip to the ER, the ICU, or worse?

What I am attempting to describe is how the "martial art" of modern MMA is essentially a set of tools with no unifying strategy: how what we have instead is a sort of hope-I-do-the-right-thing-because-I'm-so-well-versed-in-everything fatalism. But examined more closely, we see that the faith we have in this approach is largely founded on a misattribution: we see the incredible versatility of the successful modern MMA fighter and we assume that he owes his success to his versatility alone. Certainly a one-dimensional fighter will have a hard time in modern MMA, and a successful fighter needs to possess a high skill level in all areas of the fight. But to stop our consideration there is to ignore the fact that the better part of success in modern MMA hinges not on the abstract skills themselves but on the strategic application of those skills (See: Greg Jackson). Successful MMA fighters do not approach their fights with the "sharpen all the tools and see what happens" attitude. They and their team of coaches study their opponent and develop opponent-specific strategies. They spend months training specific answers to specific situations, specific counters to opponent-specific attacks (the double-leg off his opponent's consistently lazy left hook; the Muay Thai clinch off their opponent's notoriously aggressive striking style, etc.). But such specific strategizing (again: the key component of any high-level fighter's success—the success which we point to as proof of MMA as the "ultimate martial art") is only possible when that fighter 1) knows and can study his opponent, and 2) has the requisite time to develop and train the strategy designed for that opponent.

In fact, looked at more closely, we see that nearly all of the elements that comprise modern MMA (both the sport and the "martial art" that shares its name) bear the thumbprint of such sport-specific parameters. Signing a contract to fight a given opponent on a given day three months from now changes what sort of strategizing I can do, just as taping my hands and wearing gloves changes how freely and how hard I can throw punches (gloves protect the striker's hands, not the opponent's head). Knowing that I get a moment to catch my breath after five minutes of fighting gives me more freedom to push the pace. Knowing that the person I am fighting is my own weight or close to it, knowing the ref will step in to stop the action if there's a knockout, allows me to be somewhat more cavalier about stepping in and trading blows. And this is to say nothing of the myriad factors surrounding the fight: the need to deliver an "exciting fight" (read: slugfest) in hopes of gaining more fans; the need to deliver a big knockout in hopes of receiving an after-fight bonus... All of these factors alter, mutate, and confuse the incentive/disincentive system present in and inherent to a real, no-rules fight.

Or, to put it more simply: modern MMA is a sport. It is hard and it is painful and it involves kicks and punches and submissions, but it is not fighting. A cage fight with a referee and three judges and a ringside doctor is not a self-defense situation. And I say that with nothing but respect for the skill level, toughness, tenacity, etc. that these modern MMA fighters possess. I mean only that the strategy one designs for a fight with no rules, no weight classes, and no time limit must give precedence to other, and I would say more essential, priorities.

And that's exactly what Gracie Jiu-Jitsu is: not just a collection of techniques, not just a tool box full of tools, but a strategy: a manual for what, how, when, and why to apply those tools when it counts, when you're up against someone bigger, stronger, scarier, and meaner than you, when no one's going to step in to help or save you.

Like I said: I didn't always understand this. My start in Gracie Jiu-Jitsu was a little unorthodox, and was certainly limited by my own hardheadedness more than anything. Starting with the basic MMA bias (that I needed to know striking and ground fighting to be "well-rounded") and skipping as many Gracie Jiu-Jitsu classes as I attended (being that guy who only showed up for open mat, and without a gi), and seeing Steve as rarely as I did (not at all in the first two and a half years, and then only once or twice a year for the few years that followed), I never saw the forest for the trees. I learned cool moves—submissions and sweeps and chokes—but I couldn't see how they fit together into a unified theory. Worse, I thought I was looking at things with open eyes: I was an MMA guy, after all, not blinded by style loyalty or lockstep thinking hiding behind words like "respect" and "tradition."

By late 2009, however, things had changed. I was tired of leaving our weekly hard sparring sessions feeling like I couldn't do simple math, couldn't recite my own phone number, couldn't remember my own name. Most weeks I was doing my level best not to trade strikes at all: just impose the clinch, get a takedown, and apply a submission. I didn't realize that I had, in effect, defaulted into textbook Gracie Jiu-Jitsu strategy; I was just following the path of greatest success and least damage. If you had asked me at the time, I think I still might have said that this was a strategy that I liked, that worked for me, but which I was not prepared to say was better than any other. Still, by the time Steve arrived to teach a seminar in the spring of 2010, I'd almost completely forgone striking (remember, I had a black belt in a striking art!), and was spending the bulk of my MMA sparring time working it out on the ground.

At the end of that spring 2010 seminar, Steve promoted me to purple belt. I had been thrilled back in 2008 when Steve promoted me to blue belt, but purple belt put me over the moon. In my mind anybody could get a blue belt, but purple belt was something else. It was a serious rank, the halfway point between white and black belt. Afterwards Steve took me aside, and he was unequivocal about the responsibilities that rank carried. The purple belt, he told me, was like a black belt in another style: It was the rank at which you could legitimately run your own program, the rank at which you were expected to know and be able to successfully implement the core techniques and strategy of the art. I was, he said, now representing Gracie Jiu-Jitsu as a senior rank. It was on me to decide where I went from here: to decide what kind of representative I was going to be.

Honestly, up until that point, I'd thought of myself as a lot of things: a Kuk Sul Do black belt supplementing his skill set with ground fighting, an MMA guy, a grappler. I hadn't thought of myself as a representative of Gracie Jiu-Jitsu. And yet, of course, that's what I was: I was the one standing in front of the classes at The Fight Gym. I was the face of Gracie Jiu-Jitsu for anybody who walked through the door. For anyone who walked in, it would be my knowledge, my teaching ability, my skill, the things I said, my belief in the art, that would form the basis of his or her impression of Gracie Jiu-Jitsu. Wearing that belt made me an ambassador for Helio and Rickson and Royce, for the fighters and teachers I held in the highest admiration. And for Steve: Steve, who carried this same responsibility, who had put his faith in me.

Was I going to stand there and say that Gracie Jiu-Jitsu was incomplete, that it required supplements (Muay Thai, boxing, etc.), with that belt tied around my waist?

I started training Gracie Jiu-Jitsu in 2006, but I see that day in 2010 as the day that I actually started down the path to black belt. It was the day, too, that The Fight Gym stopped being a hodge-podge of disparate and often conflicting ideas and started becoming the school it is now: a school teaching and doing its level best to represent Gracie Jiu-Jitsu.

And, honestly, it has cost me students. People come to me wanting to learn boxing, kickboxing, MMA. I tell them what I do and don't teach and why, and a lot of them don't stick around. They go somewhere else to train. They know what they want to learn. They're like me back in 2006. They already know what fighting is really like, already know what really works. They watch the UFC on pay-per-view. They tell me Conor McGregor is the greatest fighter of all time. They ask me: Why don't I teach boxing? Why don't I teach Muay Thai? Isn't it better to be well-rounded?

I teach Gracie Jiu-Jitsu because I believe in Gracie Jiu-Jitsu. For those of you who are interested, I hope this post has helped you understand why I feel the way I do. For the rest of you, I hope this post has given you some ideas to consider going forward in your own practice.

I hope to see you all on the mats, very soon.

I should also say, as a final note, that nothing in this post is meant to disparage anyone's chosen style, traditional or otherwise. Whatever martial art you pursue, I hope it brings you joy and a sense of wellbeing. Training in the martial arts has brought more to my life than I can ever hope to articulate, and I wish the same for you.

VENUE
"IF GRACIE JIU-JITSU IS A COMPLETE MARTIAL ART, THEN WHY ARE YOU TRAINING JUDO?"

Originally published on JiuJitsuDoMaeda.com
May 23, 2017

Modern Judo (sport and traditional) and modern Brazilian Jiu-Jitsu (sport and traditional) both branch from the central stalk of Kodokan Judo: the stylistic differences that exist between them today are the product of the rulesets within which each has been incubating and evolving for the past hundred or so years. But return to the core art, and you find the same material: there's more similarity between Jigoro Kano's *Kodokan Judo* and Helio Gracie's *Master Text* than there is difference. So does training in Judo even "count" as training in a different style?

For the sake of argument, let's agree that it does. Even still, it's necessary to sort through the two and try to determine exactly where the distinction comes in. What makes Judo Judo and Gracie Jiu-Jitsu Gracie Jiu-Jitsu?

There are 65 throwing techniques in Kodokan Judo, and the vast majority of them are represented in the Gracie Jiu-Jitsu standing self-defense curriculum. The bulk of Gracie Jiu-Jitsu's ground techniques can be found in classical Judo. The prioritization of leverage and efficiency over strength and power comes from Kodokan Judo. Even the Gracie triangle is said to represent the three purposes of Kodokan Judo training: self-defense, physical exercise, and moral development.

So why, given these similarities, doesn't the average Judoka fight like the average Jiujiteiro?

The answer, of course, is time. The average Judo student spends the bulk of his time training on the feet, while the average Brazilian Jiu-Jitsu student spends most of his training on the ground, and the resultant differences between their skillsets represent nothing more than their greater or lesser comfort in and familiarity with different facets of an engagement. In short: The strength, effectiveness, liveliness, and adaptability of a practitioner's given technique exist in direct proportion to the amount of time that practitioner has spent attempting, failing, and refining that technique under live conditions.

So we arrive at the original question: If Gracie Jiu-Jitsu is a complete martial art, then why are you training in Judo?

Gracie Jiu-Jitsu is a complete martial art, but that does not dictate that one's training in it will automatically be complete. It is as necessary (if not more necessary: all altercations start standing) to develop live-resistance skills on the feet as it is on the ground, yet most Jiu-Jitsu students spend only a fraction of their time training either the takedowns or the standing self-defense techniques. We must understand: This is a failure of the practitioner and the training environment, *not of the art.*

So that is why I am training Judo: to give myself a venue in which to apply those aspects of the core art under live conditions. It is the same reason that, if you come to The Fight Gym for open mat, you will start every match from standing. The material is there: If the skills are lacking, then what is missing is a history of failure and refinement.

The art is complete. The art includes answers to all manner of situations. It includes takedowns, standing self-defense techniques, techniques against weapons, against strikes both standing and on the ground. The question is not: How complete is the art? The question is: How complete is your training? How often are your skills in these different areas exposed to live resistance?

Remember: A technique is just a tool. Tools are there to help us accomplish our goals more effectively, but they *don't accomplish those goals for us*. I tell my students: the hammer doesn't pound the nails, *you* pound the nails. And the success or failure of any given attempt on any given nail is going to depend a heck of a lot more on your experience with the hammer than it is on the hammer itself.

At the end of the day a dojo is just a room: just a venue. The sort of challenge you fill it with will determine the kind of skills you develop.

I wish you nothing but challenging rooms.

See you on the mats.

REPRESENT

Originally published on JiuJitsuDoMaeda.com
May 24, 2017

I met Steve Maxwell in the fall of 2008. I was 26, with a black belt in Kuk Sul Do and a couple of years' experience training Jiu-Jitsu and MMA. At that time, and though it was a big part of my life, I wasn't thinking of the martial arts as a possible career path: my not-so-secret dream was then (and had been, during and since college) to become a famous writer, the next young literary prodigy, the next F. Scott Fitzgerald or Michael Chabon, and at 26 I was still clinging to that hope, despite my mounting sense—and the mounting evidence—that it wasn't going to happen.

Steve's an interesting guy. Catch a seminar with him, or listen to him interviewed on a podcast, and you'll see what I mean. He's one of the first Americans to earn a black belt directly from the Gracies. He's one of the fathers of the American Kettlebell movement. For the better part of the last decade he's been living on the road full-time, with no home and no permanent address. He's taught seminars on fitness, mobility, kettlebells, and Gracie Jiu-Jitsu all over the country and all over the world.

In the almost ten years that I've known him, Steve has been more generous with his time and energy and knowledge than I've had any right to expect. He's taken me places I never imagined I'd go, and exposed me to things and ideas I never would have encountered if not for him. It has been an absolute privilege to spend the time with him that I have.

I wrote a novel a few years ago called *Bummed Out City*. The main character is a guy named David, a twenty-nine-year-old (mostly failed) writer with a chip on his shoulder about everything he hasn't achieved: everything the world hasn't given him. Back when I was working on it, when people would ask me what it was about, I would say, "It's about a guy who thought he was going to be a big deal writer, but isn't. He's basically me without Jiu-Jitsu."

I said it almost as a joke, but it's more true than not. Back in 2008, I was feeling pretty sorry for myself, pretty under appreciated and righteously indignant. I have to wonder where that would have ended up if it had gone unchecked.

It's common to see martial arts schools marketing their programs as a means for self-improvement and character development. Certainly anything that is challenging, that requires commitment and perseverance, can help a person develop those attributes. But in my experience nothing quite compares to Jiu-Jitsu. Feeling sorry for yourself will get you nowhere. Neither will righteous indignation, and neither will lying to or hiding from yourself. People like to say that the mats reveal you to yourself, and that's certainly been my experience. I'm not going to say the process has been particularly pleasant. I am, however, fairly convinced that it beats the alternative.

The thing that people outside the martial arts world don't necessarily understand is that a black belt is (or at least, should be) more request than accolade, more ambassador's posting than honorific title. To wear the black belt is to represent your instructor, your lineage, your art. It is to carry those responsibilities with you on and off the mat. Steve had never made a black belt before me, and getting promoted was one of the proudest days of my life, for all the reasons and in all the ways you might assume. But I have yet to tie on the belt and not feel the weight of that responsibility.

I hope that I have been and continue to be deserving of the faith that Steve has placed in me, of the time and effort he has invested in me.

If you come train with me, I promise that I will do my best to teach you what I know, to represent this art and those who have taught me.

I hope to see you all on the mats, very soon.

THE FOUR PARTS OF PERFORMANCE

Written May, 2014

This piece was written as part of an ongoing training program that I produced for a remote strength & conditioning client, who was also a Jiu-Jitsu practitioner. This piece was the first in the series.

The idea with this program is not simply to increase your work *capacity*, but also to help you develop a clearer awareness of, and more efficient use of, your work *potential*. Even if we condition you to double your work capacity, it doesn't do you much good if you go out and expend that energy in the first three minutes of a roll. For the sake of this program, then, we will consider performance as being composed of four basic parts:

1. Muscular and cardiovascular endurance
2. Mental and emotional composure
3. Leverage and efficiency
4. Effective load delegation and muscular chain recruitment

The idea here is to identify and define each of these aspects so that we can more effectively develop them as we move forward.

1. Muscular and Cardiovascular Endurance

Physical strength and endurance is the most obvious, and most seemingly straightforward, performance aspect on the list. We roll, we get out of breath, we fatigue, and we imagine that if we work out in a similar fashion (fatiguing ourselves and getting out of breath) we are helping our bodies to acclimate to the stresses of our sport while also increasing our capacity for fatiguing ourselves and getting out of breath when we engage in that sport.

There are some flaws in this approach to training (most notably this training protocol calls for heavily increasing the body's stress load, which can become a hinderance to both performance and overall health), but there is no question that some form of this approach is both necessary and effective for increasing work capacity. There are, however, a few notable and typically overlooked and underdeveloped parts of this equation that hold the potential for serious development.

I sometimes roll with people and afterwards when they're panting on the edge of the mat they'll look at me and say, "Man, I've got to work on my cardio!" I always want to ask them what they mean by this. "Cardio" is a word that is thrown around so much that no one seems to think much about what it means. Maybe the answer seems obvious: cardio means my ability to catch my breath, or not get so out of breath, right?

Well, kind of. What we're talking about when we talk about cardiovascular endurance is my body's ability to effectively supply my working muscles with oxygen (O2) while effectively eliminating carbon dioxide (CO2). This process involves three specific capacities: my heart's ability to pump my blood, my blood's ability to carry oxygen and CO2, and my lungs' ability to intake and expel air. For effective performance, each part must be working at its full potential. My heart's ability to pump my blood—i.e. cardiac strength and endurance—is (obviously) developed by forcing my heart to beat powerfully at an elevated rate for a prolonged period of time. My blood's carrying capacity for O2 and CO2 is developed by spending time in a hypo-oxygenated state (i.e. at elevation, in an elevation chamber, or under conditions in which my body's demand for oxygen stresses the limits of my ability to supply it). Training these two aspects is fairly straightforward: you train by working beyond your cardiovascular capacity (i.e. putting yourself into oxygen debt), thus prompting the body's adaptive response to improve your tolerance to these conditions.

The third component, however, is woefully misunderstood and underdeveloped in most people, even in many athletes. We tend to think that I get as much air as I get in each breath, and then it's up to my heart and my blood to do what they can with it. This is simply not the case: by understanding the physiology of breath we can absolutely train ourselves to breathe more effectively and productively, and in so doing greatly increase the amount of oxygen available to my bloodstream, while at the same time keeping my heart rate within its productive range.

Each lung is pear shaped: skinny at the top and much larger at the bottom. Accordingly, the bottom has much more surface area, and is far more vascular than the top portion. By drawing air into the lower lobes of the lungs, we effectively expose more of our blood to the air that is drawn in, resulting in much more rapid and much more efficient (molecules exchanged per breath) exchange of O2 and CO2. Drawing the air into the top portions of the lungs only, we suffer from less efficient oxygenation and waste (CO2) removal, while at the same time contributing to a state in which this problematic functioning perpetuates itself: the body doesn't get enough oxygen so it increases the heart rate in an attempt to more quickly supply oxygen to the muscles; the increased heart rate means that the blood is forced through the lungs at a faster pace, decreasing the opportunity for gas exchange, which then keeps me from effectively paying off my body's rapidly accruing oxygen debt, which causes my body to further up my heart rate, which allows for even less oxygen exchange, etc., etc. We get caught in a vicious debt cycle from which we can only escape by rapidly decreasing our fuel demands (e.g. stop working, tap out) and catch our breath.

So how do we breathe into the lower lungs? Two ways. One, we make sure we are breathing with our diaphragm. Breath works on a vacuum: the musculature of my torso expands my body cavity and creates negative air pressure. This can be accomplished in three ways: by raising my shoulders, by raising/expanding my rib cage, and by engaging my diaphragm. Of these three, the third is by far superior: only the diaphragm is specifically designed as a breathing muscle, and only diaphragmatic breathing draws the air into the lower lobes of the lungs. To keep our bodies oxygenated while performing work, it is essential that we use the diaphragm to breathe. The second way we make sure that we are breathing into the lower lungs is by inhaling only through the nose. The nose is actually rifled like a gun barrel to create a small "funnel" of air that is directed straight to the lower lobes. It is thought that it is almost impossible to effectively breathe into the lower lungs while inhaling through the mouth.

Keys to Effective Breathing Step 1: Find Your Diaphragm

Lay on your back on the floor. Put one hand on your chest and one hand on your belly button. Breathe in through the nose and exhale through the mouth. When you inhale and exhale, you should feel the hand on your belly button rise and fall. You should feel no movement in your chest. Once you're able to do this consistently and comfortably, sit up and do the same thing. You may find that, with your weight now resting on your musculoskeletal system, the process feels different. It may take some practice to do this comfortably.

Keys to Effective Breathing Step 2:"Shushing"

When you roll, attempt to keep the sensation from step one. In addition, and to help keep your focus on the breath, make your exhalation audible. Make a sound like you're "shushing" somebody. It doesn't have to be one long, continuous sound, and it doesn't always have to be the same sound. If you watch videos of Rickson rolling, you will hear him make a series of these "shushing bursts." This may get you a few weird looks in the room, but people will very quickly get used to it. The idea here is for the breath to constantly draw your own attention, to the point that you notice if an interval passes in which you make no noise (i.e. you're holding your breath) or the noise changes (you're straining). It will also help remind you that, for the time being, the breath is your first and only priority.

Allow yourself four sparring sessions to truly commit and acclimate to this new approach. You may find that, if you are previously accustomed to a more action-oriented mentality—i.e. you do what needs to be done when it needs to be done, and worry about catching your breath later—your success rate goes way down. This is to be expected. You have to consider this as essential skill-building, and your attention is going to be split. It's like running a race while trying to develop a new stride: you're not going to be competitive in the same way with the people you're used to performing well against. That's ok. This is a temporary condition, and the rewards of breathing properly—of having an optimally functioning machine—will manifest in the long run. You may find no issues, but if you do you shouldn't be discouraged by what may seem to be a decrease in your performance level.

I say to allow four sparring sessions because this type of rolling may be extremely demoralizing, and the tendency may be to abandon the approach altogether. Give it four, and then consider the experience and evaluate if you are noticing benefit. If you are definitely noticing benefit then stick with it. If you think you are noticing some benefit, but aren't sure, then give it three more sparring sessions. If you hate it and don't think it's helping and don't believe it will ever help, then we'll just stick with Approach 1.

As a side note: When I first started doing this I did it all the time, regardless of the intensity of the roll or my level of physical exhaustion. Now, I do it only in moments of fatigue or heightened stress. Blowing air from the bottom of the lungs has an immediate calming effect that in and of itself increases efficiency: i.e. you release muscular tension that is unnecessarily bleeding your oxygen supply. The point being: the idea isn't to do this forever, just until it feels natural and you are aware of your breath.

Keys to Effective Breathing Step 3: Internal Kumbhaka and Recovery Breathing

When you find that you're getting out of breath or fatigued, and you feel the impulse to switch to mouth breathing, that is when it is most important that you keep with the nasal and diaphragmatic breathing. To pay off your oxygen debt, increase the rate of your respiration (you're probably doing that already) but be sure to leave a pause between the inhalation and exhalation. This momentary holding of the breath is called *kumbhaka*, and is the moment when the gaseous exchange (the whole point of respiration, after all) occurs. If you respirate too rapidly, you expel oxygen-rich air before your body has a chance to dump its CO_2 surplus and pick up the much-needed O_2. (It need only be a momentary pause, but make sure that it's in there.)

The idea is to make this type of breathing habitual when under any physical (or even emotional) stress.

The thing to note as well about this concept of the body is that muscular function is seen largely as a product of cardiovascular function, and by improving the latter we also improve the former. The idea here is to think of the body as one integrated machine: I don't do strength work and then run for cardio; my strength work creates the oxygen demands that tax my cardiovascular system in the same way that my sport does. I will talk more about how we're going to approach our conditioning in the section on *Effective Load Delegation and Muscular Chain Recruitment*.

Action Items:

Find your diaphragm, practice diaphragmatic breathing, and then spend your next 4 sparring sessions attempting to integrate this type of breathing in your sport. If you come to a situation in which more exertion will get you a better outcome, but will also take you beyond your current breathing threshold (i.e. make you out of breath) then let it go and focus on maintaining your breath. You should never be out of breath, and you should be able to roll every round comfortably and without exhaustion. Do not expect, however, to roll to your previous level. We are setting that aside for the time being so that we may develop breathing as a skill.

2. Mental and Emotional Composure

The section on breath control and this section go hand-in-hand because, as I've mentioned, when the breath becomes the focus of the roll then performance tends to dip, in the beginning. There is a real tendency, then, to become frustrated or upset or discouraged. It is easy to be overwhelmed by these emotions when less skilled sparring partners pass my guard, etc., not due to their successful implementation of a technique but rather because I refused to "use all my juice" for fear of losing my breath. A little voice in our heads starts shouting, wanting us to tell our partner, "You didn't really pass my guard, I could have beat you if I wanted to, I'm trying this other thing, etc., etc."

Mental and emotional composure are not simply one aspect of Gracie Jiu-Jitsu: they are among the art's primary concerns. If I am fighting someone much bigger and stronger than myself, someone who has more gas in the tank, and I am unable to control my emotions, then I will be unable to control my thoughts and will be therefore unable to control my actions. I don't mean that my body will go crazy: what I mean is that, if I am unable to control my emotions, and I end up in a situation in which I can either a) remain safe in a shitty position or b) cash in all my chips to go for an unlikely escape, I am more likely to allow my irrational feeling ("I want out of here, I don't want this guy to think he's beating me, I don't want the people watching to think this guy is better than me," etc.) to decide for me, and I will pursue the improbable escape, cash in all my chips, work outside my capacity, and exhaust myself, all for an escape that was always only a semi-likely outcome (and God help me if the escape fails). If, however, I can remain in control of these feelings, if I watch them arise and understand them as my brain's natural (if unhelpful) response to these situations, and make a rational decision to wait and pursue action only when circumstances are more conducive to my success, then the probable outcome of the whole situation trends toward my success: I will go when it makes sense, when I am likely to succeed, and will stay within my work capacity in doing so.

This may seem like a small thing, but it affects every decision you make on the mat. If your true priority is energy management and conservation then there is no problem with your conditioning: you do as little as possible to stay safe, and wait for your opponent to tire. This is Helio Gracie Jiu-Jitsu. I often tell people: It's not about how much gas you have in the tank, it's about how you use the gas that you have.

The heart of the problem is *want*. When we want things—when we allow that emotion to color and distort our reason—then we pursue irrational paths. Imagine that you have a dog: you lock this dog in its crate, and you set a hamburger just outside the door. The dog will whine and scratch and claw at the gate; it will press its nose to the bars and stick its tongue through trying in vain to reach the hamburger. It will exhaust itself pursuing a goal it will never, ever achieve. We like to think of ourselves as being smarter than a dog, and yet many of us use this same caliber of thinking: in the midst of an action-packed roll, we see the object of our desire (a transition or submission we think we can get) and it feels so very close that we go for it without a second thought.

Sometimes our attempts are successful, and sometimes they are not. Almost invariably, however, they are a fight: we haven't cleared the path, haven't neutralized our opponent's ability to oppose us, and so we're left trying to fight our way through some form of the dog crate. Maybe we make it through and get the hamburger, maybe we don't, but definitely, one way or the other, we are "dog" tired at the end of it.

If we can learn to let go—or at least become suspicious—of want (the overwhelming and insistent and visceral and excitable feeling), then there is never any cause to pursue a course that will take me beyond my work capacity. I call it "doing the math": you consider the situation without desire or investment, and you pursue the course that makes sense based on the criteria prescribed (energy conservation, natural body movements, muscular efficiency, skeletal framing, etc.). I will address this more in the next section on *Leverage and Efficiency*, but that section requires that we develop the detachment that composure affords us.

The word "ego" is thrown around a lot in Jiu-Jitsu academies, and people will often (irony of ironies) pridefully proclaim that they "have no ego," that they "leave their ego at the door," that they'll "tap to anybody." These people have no fucking idea what they're talking about. To understand ego, you have to understand that its primary emotion is want. I *want* to be seen a certain way. I *want* to beat this person, and feel good about myself. I *want* to get this submission. I *want* to pass the guard. I *want* to escape the side control. I don't *want* to be beat by this person. I don't *want* people to think x, y, or z about me.

This is not a question of reorienting your hoped-for outcome. The goal is always to win. This is a question of ending our emotional relationship with winning. Our emotions excite and agitate and eventually exhaust us. Not having an ego means not allowing the irrational, emotional self to run the show. It means looking at what is in front of you without desire or attachment.

Watch, the next time you roll. Let someone less skilled than yourself have a good position on you, and create a situation in which they think they're going to submit you. Watch their demeanor change. Listen to their breath rate increase. Feel the tension come into their body. They want that submission so bad! Then, when you escape, watch how exhausted they are. That is the ego running the show: the entirely forgivable and entirely human and, finally, entirely stupid operating system we're all born with. Your job is to use intelligence to win, not desire.

So how do we forgo and transcend the ego? Well, for one thing, we don't. Not in any sustainable way. Monks spend their entire lives with only this goal in mind, and when they succeed it's called enlightenment. Are we going to become enlightened doing this a few minutes a day, as a hobby? Probably not. But we can develop and employ and strengthen the ego-management skills the monks use, and sustain a state of ego-suspension for the duration, at least, of a roll.

The method is to watch your thoughts as they arise, recognize that they are only suggestions, and allow them to fade back into nothingness. Sit completely still for four minutes. And by completely still, I mean completely still. Don't shift your weight. Close your eyes and don't open them. Don't flare your nostrils. Don't scratch your head. This should be easy at first, and rapidly become extremely uncomfortable. Since you cannot move, you must watch the gymnastics your mind starts to perform: you will want to stop, will want to move. Your brain will start to convince you that what you've already done is enough, that it's ok to move now. Your brain will start to convince you that I, Scott, don't know what I'm talking about, that I don't know about your bad knee or your back problems, and that

that changes the rules. It will try to convince you that this whole thing is unreasonable. Your job is to sit there and watch these thoughts come into your head, shout and protest, and then go out again.

The next day, do it for five minutes. Increase one minute every day until you reach twelve minutes. After you've reached twelve minutes, go to the gym and find the biggest guy there and have him put you in side control. Escape ONLY when the path is clear and easy. If you have to use more than 30% of your power and energy, stop trying to escape. Attempt to watch your thoughts in the same way you did when you were sitting still. Your brain will try to trick you in the same way, into doing things that don't make pure, rational sense. The goal is to be smarter than your brain.

Once you've done that, the next phase is to induce fear. After all: there are no real consequences when we're sitting in a room, and the worst thing that can happen in the gym is me getting tapped.

You can use a jump rope, or just jog in place. Take a full inhale, then exhale all the air out of your lungs and hold your breath (this is called *external kumbhaka*). With your breath held, start skipping rope or jogging in place. When you can't stand it any longer (usually this will be accompanied by an involuntary swallowing action in the throat), stop running or skipping rope and take one nasal inhale, exhale fully, hold your breath again, and resume activity. Obviously each *external kumbhaka* will be shorter and shorter, but the goal of the exercise is to, despite the panic, retain control of yourself sufficiently to enforce the kumbhaka, if only for a moment. Do this for ten breaths, then rest (but be sure to recover with nasal inhale and diaphragmatic breathing).

This should be really, really unpleasant. You may notice, however, that afterwards rolling just doesn't seem that bad.

Action Items:

- Sit completely still for four minutes, and increase the time spent sitting still daily until you are sitting completely still for twelve minutes.

- Start in the bottom of side control against a large opponent, and refuse to pursue any escape that requires more than 30% effort.

- Perform light aerobic activity with *external kumbhaka*.

3. Leverage and Efficiency

Leverage is one of those words like "base" and "ego": it gets used a lot, but most people don't seem to have a good working definition for what it means. In its simplest form, and for the purposes of this discussion, leverage means: the ability to create force in a given direction superior to the force that can be offered in opposition. For example: If I pull on your wrist with both hands, I have leverage because my ability to move that wrist toward myself is greater than your ability to pull it toward yourself.

Breaking it down simply, all efforts within a given engagement fall into one of three categories with regards to their effect: 1) the input/effort is greater than the output/effect (inefficient), 2) the input/effort is equal to the output/effect (efficient), and 3) the input/effort is less than the output/effect (greater and greater efficiency).

Our discussion is going to focus on the first two categories, and leave the third for a later date.

Baseline mechanical efficiency, then, means that for every unit of energy I put into a situation I create an accompanying comparable effect in a 1:1 ratio. Meaning that if I push your shoulder an inch and it moves an inch I am efficient. None of the push is lost between input and output. Compare that to the common situation in which I push you hard enough to move your shoulder an inch and it only moves half an inch, because you create an opposing force, requiring me to input twice as much energy to create the same effect, throughout which my input is less than my effect.

Greater mechanical efficiency affords us better outcomes (situation to situation, and overall) while also decreasing our energy expenditure. Combine this with the work demand (the one-inch push I'm trying to create) being spread across multiple work systems (the body working in concert, not simply my arm pushing your arm) and we create a situation in which we have consistent energy output that falls well within our work capacity (again: it's not just about how much gas I have in the tank, it's about how I use the gas that I've got).

The better part of situational leverage, however, is more subtle than the two-on-one example. Every pass, every transition, every move and counter is a small battle for leverage, and even though we all know this, I think very few of us stop and think about what it really means on a micro-moment-to-micro-moment level. In order to do that, we have to look a little closer at the mechanics of leverage.

Leverage is a question of innate physical functionality. The human body works and doesn't work in certain fairly universal ways. Some of these are obvious, and form what we think of as the core of BJJ, e.g. my elbow doesn't bend past 180 degrees. Some of them are less obvious, and often get overlooked. For example: my ability to contract my tricep (i.e. move my hand away from my shoulder) is greatest when the angle at my elbow is between 45 and 135 degrees. My ability decreases as I reach the extremes of the range of motion (my ability to extend from 0 to 45 and from 135 to 180). If you, as my opponent, force my arm to work within this weaker range of motion (by staying too tight in side control for me to move my forearm more than 45 degrees off my upper arm) you can then easily maintain a leverage advantage due not to your relative strength but to my relative weakness.

It is important here to note that we are making a distinction between innate physical functionality (the way the proper alignment of my muscles and joints can produce effect, the way strength through any given range of motion falls along a bell curve) and conditioned physical ability (my working up to a 400-hundred-pound bench press). While it is true that strengthening a given movement pattern will increase force potential across the entire range of motion, the question of relative strength still remains paramount: if I am able to bench press 400 through the middle part of the movement pattern, but am only able to recruit a minority percentage of that potential force because my arm is forced to work in an inefficient and mechanically disadvantageous position, my opponent's relative advantage will overcome my conditioned physical ability.

To discover relative leverage, then, we have to form a working catalogue of the body's primary movement patterns.

I often say that my body is basically good at doing two things: pulling me into the fetal position and extending me out of the fetal position. All of my muscles and joints basically align and function to facilitate these two gross body movements. If we break this down a bit more, we can further divide these two major movement patterns into five specialized movement patterns. These are:

1. Vertical Push/Vertical Pull (push/pull overhead, force in line with the spine)

2. Lateral Push/Lateral Pull (push/pull in front of the body, force perpendicular to the spine)

3. Lower body anterior-side dominant extension (pushing the feet away from the hips)

4. Lower body posterior-side dominant extension (erecting the body from a bent-at-the-waist position)

5. Stabilization and rotation of the spine

These five movement patterns, when performed correctly, involve every major muscle group as well as the connective tissues between muscle groups (muscular chains). This estimation of the body forms the basis of the workouts I create for Fight Gym students, and should form the basis of the criteria through which you view your Jiu-Jitsu. Movements made within these movement patterns are innately strong because they are the movements our anatomy is designed to produce; when we use our bodies in this manner while forcing our opponent's body to work in positions and ranges of motion that fall outside of these parameters, we effectively produce and maintain a leverage advantage. True, there is some variation across the spectrum when it comes to conditioned mechanical ability, e.g. if I put my opponent in an Americana from side control, and my opponent is able to chest fly 300 pounds, he will be able to produce considerable force in opposition to my submission attempt; however, if I am orienting my body properly, engaging through the legs and torso in opposition to this force, I still have dominant leverage.

This is one of the key considerations when it comes to the question of conditioning, because fatigue is accelerated by—and often, in fact, prompted by—inefficient mechanics. Take the previous example of the Americana from side control: if I am on the bottom, and I attempt to escape the Americana by bringing my arm in front of my body, I may or may not escape depending on my opponent's effective use of his position. Regardless of this, however, such inefficient use of my body will demand a large input of energy, and leave me needing to catch my breath and recover. If, however, I turn and face my arm and draw my elbow back toward my body (in basically a vertical pull motion), my motion is both stronger and easier, giving me greater effectiveness while requiring less energy.

Arguably, this previous example is a question of technique. But take another, simpler example. I am facing an opponent on the feet. I am pushing him, and he is pushing me. If I orient my body somewhat sideways, so that my rear kneecap is pointing out, the connective tissues that bind the exterior side of my knee and ankle are being forced to work against the force being applied against me by my opponent. If, however, I turn my leg so that my knee is facing my opponent and the ball of my foot is engaged with the floor, similar to how I might stand if I was getting ready to run a sprint, my muscles and joints work to bear and oppose the force being directed against them.

Again, this is a question of micro-moment to micro-moment adjustments which, over the course of a five or ten or twenty minute fight have a cumulative effect on my overall work demand.

The word we are circling here is *alignment*. When I bring my body into proper alignment I am able to transfer force from one muscle group and movement pattern to the next to produce an overall effect that is sustainable, efficient, and mechanically greater than the sum of the force produced by any one of the constituent parts. When you are sparring and or working out, I encourage you to think in terms of loading weight and creating force along your body's innate movement "tracks."

The other thing I haven't mentioned is that this approach, when applied correctly and consistently, greatly reduces your chance of injury on the joints and connective tissues. The joint must be strained beyond its normal range of motion, or the muscle pushed beyond its normal elongation, to produce damage; by actively aligning our movement patterns we greatly reduce the likelihood of a force being applied to our joints or muscles when they are positioned in a moment of mechanical weakness.

Action Items:

While sparring, think about facing your opponent directly at all times. Set this as the primary condition that must be met before any "move" or action is attempted.

4. *Effective Load Delegation and Muscular Chain Recruitment*

You can think of this section as a continuation of the previous section. Here is where we get into some specifics.

Effective load delegation means placing the burden of the work across all of the muscle groups involved in the movement pattern being employed. This is a matter of degree, because it is of course impossible to perform any movement pattern without all of the constituent parts being employed to some degree (the movement wouldn't succeed). It is possible, however, to under-load one part of the chain while over-loading another. It is also possible to time my movements in such a way that the weakest parts of the chain are only engaged once the load is in motion, i.e. when the force working on the load has made it "lighter" (i.e. if I have to pick something heavy up off the floor in a dead lift motion, and I create an explosive upward lift with my lower back before engaging my hamstrings, the load on my hamstrings will be lighter than the load on my lower back due to the upward force, generated by my lower back, working momentarily on the load). For the purposes of motor skill learning and conditioning we want to avoid these "cheats" at all costs. As such, all reps of exercises working the 5 basic movement patterns should be performed slowly and as smoothly as possible through the entire range of motion.

Basically, the point of working these 5 movement patterns is to 1) develop strength across the entire range of motion while 2) learning a basic motor skill (the ability to effectively concert muscle group actions against a load). The point should almost never be to hit an arbitrary "goal" number of reps, or perform the given reps within a set time. When it comes to the exercises that load the 5 basic movements patterns, I never have my students perform sprinting reps. Remember that the real definition of "cardio" is my body's ability to effectively supply oxygen to working muscles; performing workouts that mimic the work I will be asking my body to do while rolling affords me a fantastic opportunity to develop the skill of cardiovascular function.

What follows is a breakdown of the main exercises I have my Fight Gym students do, with explanations of what we want to think about when we're performing them. Again, all of these exercises should be performed smoothly (no "bouncing" to start the motion at the top or bottom) and at a slow, even pace.

The Vertical Push, i.e. the overhead press. My favorite way to train this is with the dive bomber push-up (or sometimes a limited variation, the pike push-up or "down-dog" push-up). There is a real tendency to flare the elbows when performing the overhead press, putting the lats at a disadvantage and placing the load on the shoulder joint. We want to avoid this. To do the dive bomber push-up: start in downward-facing dog with your elbows pointed out to the sides and your shoulders shrugged up by your ears. Begin the motion by bending the elbows, rotating the points of the elbows back and the pit of the elbow forward, engaging the lats and drawing the shoulders down the back (away from the ears), as you do. Continue to lower yourself down and forward until your nose is almost touching the floor between your hands. Your upper arms should now be tight against your rib cage. Continue the forward motion, dropping your hips toward the floor and lifting your head as you extend the arms (elbow points rotating out), and glide through into upward-facing dog. Reverse the motion exactly as it was performed going forward, keeping your elbows snug to your sides at the bottom position and rotating the elbows out as you extend. The last quarter of the motion—from the low push-up position into downward-facing dog, will be the most difficult part.

You can also isolate the vertical push aspect of the exercise by performing only the first and the fourth sections, i.e. moving from downward-facing dog until your nose touches the floor between your hands, and then pushing back again (pike push-up or "down-dog push-up"). This is in some ways superior because, as your spine is not forced to articulate to facilitate the "diving through" motion, you can more easily and more consistently engage your lower back through the whole motion, and in particular the pressing phase. This is important, as a true overhead press relies heavily on the underlying structures (the torso and legs), in particular the erecting function of the posterior chain. In light of this, it is also advantageous to work the overhead press from a standing position using a weight.

The Vertical Pull. Among vertical pull exercises, the pull-up is the undisputed king. Grip the bar with hands at shoulder width. Begin the motion by trying to break the bar in half as you would a stick: engage through the hands and wrists, rotate the points of the elbows forward, engage the lats, pull the shoulders down the back and pinch them together around your spine (you should start to tilt back like you're doing a front lever). Attempt to touch your Adam's apple (or even your sternum) to the bar. As you do, imagine that you are trying to connect the knobs on the inside of your elbows to your floating ribs on either side. Do this for a few weeks, and then let somebody try to get your arms away from your sides in mount.

Once you feel like your pull-up is really clean, then it's time to make it even more effective. From a dead hang, do a slight crunch. Rotate your pelvis like you're tucking your tail between your legs. Curve your lower back slightly. Now do your pull-up. If you're doing this right, it should be significantly harder. The idea here is to imagine your vertical pull as an entire front-side movement: I'm not just pulling with my arms, I'm trying to take whatever I'm holding (in this case, the bar) and pull it with me as I tuck into the fetal position.

The Lateral Push. If you put 50 people in a room and asked them each to do a push-up, you would probably get 50 different versions of what a push-up looks like. Some people just have terrible form because they don't know any better. Some people have terrible form because they read something once talking about the supposed benefits of the way they're doing their push-ups. The version of the push-up that I do is concerned with two things: safety and functionality. The safety aspect we already talked about in the section on the dive bomber push-up, but the functionality aspect merits some further discussion.

Imagine (or actually go do this) that you're pushing a wall. The engagement isn't just going to be in your arms, or your arms and chest, or even your arms and chest and abs. Pushing something (a wall, a boulder, another person) on the feet is an entire anterior-side engagement. When we do our push-ups, however, most of us are content to work the arms and pectorals and call it good.

Get into the push-up position, palms on the floor directly beneath the shoulders. Come up onto the very tips of your toes, and then try to push your toes through the ground. Literally imagine that you're at the beach and you are trying to drive them further and further into the sand. You should feel your abs light up right away but if you don't, the next step will get them: pinch your butt cheeks together and tuck your tailbone between your legs (this should create a slight "hollow" in your belly and a slight bulge in the lower back). Now drop your sternum toward the floor without bending your arms (i.e. allow your shoulders to drop behind you) and pinch your shoulder blades together around your spine. If you're doing this correctly, you should almost have that "over the top" feeling you get on the first hill on a roller coaster: you should feel like your weight is shifted ever so slightly forward, like you're about to tip forward. Now lower yourself to the floor, keeping the same engagement through the legs and core. Touch the nose to the floor, then allow the curve in your lower back to relax and touch your chest between your hands. Recreate the hollow, tucking your tailbone and engaging the abs, and start to extend the arms. If you're doing this right, it will feel like doing a push-up with a weight plate on your back.

This is the most function-oriented push-up I've found, and will not only develop your strength but will also develop your whole-body engagement sensibility, which again is one of the keys to efficient work (distributing the force burden over numerous muscular systems).

The Lateral Pull. This should be performed as basically the exact opposite motion of the lateral push. For this, I don't think there's a better exercise than the bodyweight row. A TRX, or a set of low gymnastic rings, is perfect for this. Start with your feet directly beneath the anchor point. Think about pressing your heels into the floor in the same way you pressed your toes into the floor on the previous exercise. Arch your back (belly slightly pressed forward) and engage the posterior chain (hamstrings, gluteals, and lower back). Start with the elbows pointing out and away from each other. Rotating the elbow points down and the pits of the elbows forward as you row. Draw your shoulders down your back and toward each other, pinching your spine. Elbows should scrape the sides as you pull your chest between the rings. Make sure you move slowly, as it is very easy to use momentum on this exercise to carry you through the weaker parts of the range of motion, in particular the very top.

Lower body Anterior-Side-Dominant Extension. In terms of functionality and simplicity, I love the simple bodyweight squat. Start with your feet shoulder width apart, toes pointing forward, feet running parallel to one another. Keeping your back straight and your torso upright, lower yourself down, allowing the knees to come forward but keeping the heels on the ground. You want to be able to sit all the way down until your hips are touching your heels. This is of paramount importance in BJJ, where my legs must be strong through the full range of motion, and must be comfortably able to accommodate the more extreme end of the range of motion. If you find that you are unable to perform the full depth bodyweight squat, you must prioritize working into it. An easy way is to hold onto something for balance as you perform the squat (most people find that their lack of flexibility causes them to tip over backwards). Whatever loss of load comes from the assist is mitigated by the benefit gleaned from working the full range of motion. Again, do not bounce at the bottom of the motion, and in particular make sure that the shoulders are over the hips (torso is upright) when you are extending out of the down position (the tendency is to let the hips rise while bending forward, greatly reducing the load demand on the front thighs). Exhale into the squat, inhale when you return to standing.

Lower body Posterior-Side-Dominant Extension. This is, I think, the most overlooked and under-developed part of most people's training, and is of absolutely paramount importance for Jiu-Jitsu practitioners. Want a ridiculously heavy open guard? Want to never get stacked in an arm bar or triangle again? Develop and utilize your posterior chain.

There are two exercises that are fantastically good at developing the posterior chain, and one is about as good as the other (you can almost use them interchangeably in a workout): the kettlebell swing and the dead lift. When I do either, I must absolutely make sure that I am not allowing the front thighs to take over the motion.

For either exercise, do the following movement pattern drill. Stand with feet shoulder width or slightly wider, feet running parallel and toes pointed forward. Pack your shoulders (give yourself a big, "superhero" chest), arch your lower back (stick your butt out like a posturing ape) and bend over at the waist, allowing the hips to drop back. Knees should bend, but the kneecaps should not come forward. Shins should stay dead vertical. Allow your arms to rotate in the shoulder socket and find the plumb line (the vertical line off the shifting line of your torso). Arms should run parallel to and only slightly in front of your shins. Once your fingers touch your feet or the ground, depending on the width of your stance, engage your gluteals and force your hips forward, using the engagement in your lower back to direct the push all the way up your spine. At the top you should feel engagement through the lower back, glutcals, and hamstrings.

This is the hinge: the posterior-side dominant bend and extension. The dead lift should be exactly this motion. The kettlebell swing, obviously, requires more movement in the arms, but the motion with the hips should be exactly the same. With the kettlebell swing, it is absolutely essential that the hips generate the motion: hips catch the arms and drop back, hips push the arms and propel them forward (it is the swinging of the arms that translates the motion up; there is no real upward lift with the hips themselves).

Stabilization and Rotation of the Spine. Honestly, I don't even do devoted "core exercises" anymore. What more functional engagement would an isolation exercise produce than what we're doing in our push-up, pull-up, row, etc.? If you are doing these properly, then your core is getting plenty of work, and not just the cosmetic stuff that most people do, but real, functional chain engagement that will help you recruit the core for the work it's designed to do (translating a push or pull from the feet through the arms, etc.).

Again, these movement patterns form the core of my conditioning focus, and accordingly these half-dozen or so exercises comprise the main ingredients of the workouts I create for my students.

WANTING OUTCOMES

Written June, 2014
This piece was written as part of an ongoing training program that I
produced for a remote strength & conditioning client, who
was also a Jiu-Jitsu practitioner.

The Buddhists say that desire is the root of all suffering, and this is never more evident than on the Jiu-Jitsu mat: push for something that just isn't quite there, some move that just isn't going to happen, and chances are you end up worse off than when you started, and gassed to boot.

While it is sometimes a manageable task to resign ourselves at the outset to failure and/or self-denial (i.e. "I'm rolling with ____, so I'm definitely going to get tapped somehow"; "There are always cookies at mom's house, but I've already decided that I'm not going to eat any cookies"), it's another thing altogether to let go of our attachment to the outcomes we have almost achieved, the ones that feel achingly close (the Kimura that's almost there; the cookie that's already on its way to your mouth).

Sure, it sucks that guys who are better than you beat you, but you may have found that you don't get as exhausted rolling with those guys: you're already familiar (i.e. "comfortable") with the outcome.

It's the people who are right at your level—the ones on whom you're not sure a pass or a submission is going to work, who you're not sure you can tap, where the match could go either way—that really get the heart pumping.

What I am talking about is those moments where our desire for a specific outcome—and our anxiety about achieving it—drive us to use excess speed and/or force, where our adrenaline response is triggered and we feel the physiological uplift and the crash that follows. The irony, of course, is that the faster and harder we go, and the more anxious we become, the less present and sensitive we become to the nuances of the position, and the more likely we are to fail (prompting us to have even more anxiety the next time we're in that situation with that partner...).

Even in the Buddha's time, there was some confusion about his teachings: How was it possible to desire nothing? Was the goal a sort of austerity, a profound self-denial, a living death? Was it to act as one's own vigilant watchman, constantly denying one's own impulses? Was it to retreat from the world and see in it only a passing and vapid pageant (and to ever deny one's own ever-recurring impulse to engage with it)?

I wrote a blog post not too long ago about the nature of worry, its function in our lives, and what happens to us when we use this "tool" too often. The upshot of the whole thing was this: that we feel a sort of visceral attachment to the things we care about, and we often channel this emotional energy into fantasies of disaster (we move from "I love this person/thing" to "What would happen if this person/thing went away?"). This is the mechanism of worry. We do this so fluidly and so constantly that some of us are unable to delineate the boundary between love and worry. Yet the two are fundamentally different, both philosophically and emotionally: love is delight in the present; worry is fear of the (potential) future. By allowing ourselves to feel or express our love as worry we take ourselves out of the moment, we wash ourselves in the negative hormone cascade that accompanies fear, and we poison the relationship with the person/thing we love by interacting with it in a negative way.

There is an alternative, which is difficult not only because most of us are out of practice but also in and of itself, and that is to (almost paradoxically) remain fully invested (emotionally and intellectually) in the present, yet fully disinterested in any outcome. If we can do this, we can maintain a state of relaxation and openness, and avoid the negative physiological effects of the stress that comes with fear of, or anxiety about, the future.

This is great in life in general, but this is also a super productive way to be on the mat: be totally present and mindful, but totally disinterested in the outcome of any given roll. And that doesn't mean: "I don't care if I tap." It means I'm not giving any of my thought energy to imagining an outcome, good or bad. I am not resigned to success or failure, I am not trying to pretend that I don't get butterflies in my stomach when I think I'm going to hit a submission on a guy I've never submitted before. I am actively thinking of every situation and every exchange as another word in a monotone sentence—there are no shouts, there are no exclamation points, it's all just the same, moment to moment to moment.

So, how in the hell do we develop that?

Before I get into it, I should mention that I am absolutely not awesome at this. What I am saying is: this is a skill (albeit an intangible thought skill) that, just like throwing a ball or riding a bike, we can develop and strengthen by practice. Plenty of people still provoke me out of my little "Zen" state. Go a little bit too hard at me, act like a jackass, etc., and my mind starts turning, thinking of how I want to teach you a lesson and how great it's going to be when I do. Similarly, if I meet a tough purple belt or even a tough blue belt, and he starts giving me trouble, my mind starts running with fearful thoughts: "This guy's only a blue belt, I'm supposed to be way better than him, what if he taps me," etc., etc. Once I started paying attention to my own thoughts, however, I began to notice how these thoughts alone were enough to elevate my heart rate and change my breathing—were enough to make me exhibit the signs and symptoms of fatigue even in the absence of an increased physical demand.

To counter this, I started considering this as the worst possible outcome of a roll: not tapping, but losing my mental composure.

There were a couple of key related realizations that had to come along with this, and the first was the acceptance that anyone can be tough. Being a white belt does not mean you're weak, that you have no athletic ability, that you aren't smart enough to figure out what's going on. It would be great if we, being higher belts, were so much better that we just embarrassed everyone who ever came in the door, but it just doesn't work like that. Helio used to say, "A strong guy is born with Jiu-Jitsu," meaning that a guy who is strong is endowed with tools that he may use to persevere in a physical confrontation. Knowing Jiu-Jitsu doesn't mean that I'm going to easily knock everybody down: it means that I have the tools to manage anybody I encounter. And that is realization number two: that the goal here is to have the tools to *manage* a confrontation with anyone. If I go in expecting to dominate and murder everyone I'm not only setting myself up for frustration, I am also expressly misunderstanding what Jiu-Jitsu is.

So, step one: take nothing for granted. Assume that anyone, no matter their belt, has the tools necessary to hurt you. Once you accept this, you no longer have to feel that your ego is being threatened when a strong guy is strong with you. He's strong: what does a belt have to do with it? Deal with the problem at hand. Don't worry about "how it looks" that some blue belt is giving the brown belt a run for his money. (The other thing to remember is that this—treating the blue belt as your peer—is the only viable option for success; the other option is to try to "put him in his place," which will most commonly result in over-exertion, frustration, over-adrenalization, etc.)

Step two: pursue your objective as a matter of course. Don't try to *make* anything happen. Take things when they are easy to take. If you get mounted, don't bump like crazy to escape. Defend the arms and the chokes, and work your leg flat to the ground. Once the leg is flat, make your frame. Once you've made your frame, start to work the escape. Let each piece of the escape open the door to the next piece. If you get stopped or countered at any point, then go back and start over. Don't let frustration or anxiety—or a vision of what *might* happen—overwhelm you. Recognize that you, as a person in a confrontation, want certain outcomes, and that with that desire will come frustration. Acknowledge that your brain is doing this, and then recognize that your frustration is not a helpful aspect of your thought process, and recommit yourself to the task at hand. Think about an ant trying to carry something up a hill: if he gets stopped, he doesn't stand there bitching about how unfair or annoying it is, he doesn't cling to what he hoped would happen, how he thought things would go. He just moves forward where he can. He is involved in the minute adjustments required by the course immediately in front of him. He knows where he's going: he doesn't need to wish to go there, hope that he can get there, or become frustrated when he isn't there yet. He doesn't waste energy with useless thoughts—thoughts that are not helping him achieve his objective.

So: when you're rolling (or really, when you're doing anything) and you find yourself frustrated by a task (because you thought it was going to be easy, because you thought it would only take 5 minutes, because you thought you'd be done in time for ____), recognize the appearance of this frustration, recognize the frustrated desired outcome at the end of it, recognize that fear and anxiety are the product of the disparity between present reality and potential future, and then let go of that potential future. You can literally envision it floating off into space until it disappears. Once you do that you will find that your attention refocuses on the task at hand (you no longer have one foot in the room and one foot out the door), and the outcome will come to you on its own.

For the next month, your rolling mantra is: mindfulness in the present produces the desired result; mindfulness of the desired result sabotages both the present and the result.

It is anxiety—the desire for or against a potential outcome, and our uncertainty about it—that causes a great deal of our fatigue via over-exertion and adrenaline response. The idea is to acknowledge and relinquish your attachment not to the outcome (obviously we still want to beat the guy), but to the appearance of the outcome as a part of my mental process (the vision we have of the potential outcome). These thoughts—these concerns about a future state—draw us out of our engagement with the present moment in all things, but very tellingly on the Jiu-Jitsu mat, where not being in the moment can have immediate negative repercussions. So when you find yourself envisioning an outcome, let that vision go. If you can successfully implement this, I think you'll find that this, more than anything else, greatly affects your level of both exertion and fatigue when rolling.

IDENTIFY YOUR INFLECTION POINTS

Written July, 2014
This piece was written as part of an ongoing training program that I
produced for a remote strength & conditioning client, who
was also a Jiu-Jitsu practitioner.

"Jiu-Jitsu is perfect. It's humans who make errors."

—Master Rickson Gracie

The human brain is a marvel of efficiency. Any repeated movement, behavior, situation-specific response, etc. becomes more automatic and (mentally) effortless with each subsequent repetition. If you've ever watched a child grow from infancy to toddlerhood, then what you've watched is a process by which a series of uncoordinated movements slowly concert themselves, slowly become locomotion, speech, and higher and higher motor skills. You've seen how much concentration those first steps took, and have watched how—with repetition—that movement took less and less effort. The hundreds of tiny coordinations that have to happen so that one foot bears the weight while the other lifts simply becomes a bundle called "taking a step."

As an infant, your brain is learning (through a protracted period of almost ceaseless trial and error) the precise series of muscular engagements that produce useful action. Once that pattern is learned, however, your brain no longer has to actively perform each part. Instead, it goes on pre-programmed auto-pilot: It's more like your brain is saying, "Ok, initiate the 'take a step' sequence," and your body just follows its programming. And with each step you take, that programming gets more and more embedded and more and more efficient.

Or, just as relevantly—think about the hip-away. The first time you did it you had to think about a hundred different things; now, if I tell you to do a hip-away, you just do the whole thing without much thought. This is how the brain works: a complicated series of movements and behaviors becomes a programmed bundle.

This is one of the truly amazing things about the human brain, but it can also be one of the most disastrous. Ever heard the maxim that practice makes permanent? This mental faculty means that any repeated behavior becomes more habitual, stronger, and harder to break, and this can really screw us up when we don't like the outcomes that a given behavior pattern is producing (at the far extreme end of the spectrum, think addiction). Despite an awareness of the negative consequences of a given behavior, individuals may find themselves (nearly) powerless to override their programming.

We started off talking about bundles related to physical engagement (i.e. stepping and shrimping), but the same phenomenon occurs with intangible behaviors. Ever had a friend, coworker, or casual acquaintance with whom you couldn't *not* argue? Even though you knew you would leave the exchange feeling bad, somehow as soon as you got around them, they just brought it out in you? Or maybe you know someone who, whenever the stakes are high at work or recreation (maybe at BJJ), performs below their demonstrated ability. They may even say later, "I don't know what it is. I know what I'm supposed to do, but every time I get in there and I'm staring at the prize, I blow it."

These are also programmed bundles: they are patterns of responses (emotional, verbal, physical, physiological) associated with specific stimuli. Once a cue is sounded (the boss hands the presentation over to us; the girl seems to be enjoying the date; the ref asks me if I'm ready) a chain of small decisions starts, and we cruise down the path we've programed into our brains.

Once we're down one of these programming paths, it's almost impossible to get out of it. It's like karaoke—you picked a song you thought was going to be funny, but once you start singing it no one laughs, and now you've got to stick it out until the end. The secret to correcting this bad programming is not to tweak the program but to write an entirely new program for that situation, and that starts with identifying the inflection point.

The inflection point is the initial cue, the trigger that sets us off into our programming. It doesn't have to be all external, nor does it have to be general. Rather, our programming tends to be very situation specific. Let me give you an example:

A couple years ago (I had just received my brown belt) a specific episode started cropping up in my Jiu-Jitsu life. I would go somewhere for an open mat and a white or a blue belt would ask to roll with me (guys around here don't get the whole "don't ask a higher belt to roll" thing). I would go in to roll, just to go light and warm up, and those guys would go apeshit. I would get annoyed, and start to fight them back (giving a lot of strength and energy output). My effectiveness would go way down, my technique would go to shit, and my breathing and composure would go right out the window. I would finish the roll feeling bad about myself and my skill set, annoyed with the guy for rolling like a jackass, and wanting to just leave and be done with training for the day.

This happened more than once. It happened often enough that I started being able to identify certain features of these episodes. The features weren't always present, but they usually were.

I didn't know the person who was asking to roll with me. Often it was their or my first time at the school.

I was tired. I was training out of habit. I didn't particularly want to go to the gym, but I went anyway because I didn't want to not go.

I had other stuff on my mind. I don't mean that there was something hanging over my head. I mean that, when I stopped to pay attention, I could see that my thoughts were somewhere else.

I had an unrealistic expectation of how the guy was going to train. There was a disconnect between what we each thought was happening. I was thinking of the roll as a warmup; he was thinking of it as a personal test.

When the guy started getting strong and explosive with me, I let myself feel superior and indignant about it (i.e. "This guy's a fucking jackass"). That made me feel like I was justified in going outside my comfort zone ("I'm going to go hard, and show this guy who he's messing with!") and inevitably either 1) left me more frustrated and tired when my attempts didn't work, or 2) kept me from feeling good about whatever outcome I'd achieved, since I'd muscled it.

So: a specific situation (the whole scenario, with all of its internal and external factors, is my inflection point) sets off a chain of behaviors, decisions, and perceptions that lead to negative outcomes.

So what do we do about this? The real problem with inflection points is that our brain is so good at efficiently kicking into our programming that we're often already down the path before we know what hit us. However, once we recognize our inflection points, we can start to anticipate them and pre-make the decision about what our first response is going to be. Think about the smoker who, when he feels the need to smoke, eats a carrot. Or the alcoholic in recovery who, when he goes to a cookout where people are drinking, brings his own case of soda. Once we start down a new path, we can either link up with other programming (the pitcher who does great in practice but chokes in the game, is able to link up with the practice habits, etc.) or forge (as the infant learning to walk) new programming that will, with trial and error, become a new bundle.

For the inflection point I described for myself, the solution was to either 1) decline their request to roll, or 2) go in expecting a fight, and play a tight, conservative game.

And so the quote at the beginning of this essay: Jiu-Jitsu itself may be complete and perfect, but when funneled through my anxiety, stress, and frustration, and the poor decision-making that comes with all three, it comes out looking nothing like itself. If I can identify those inflection points that cause me to become a (more) imperfect expression of the art, however, I can more effectively avoid those negative outcomes associated with poor execution.

THE REAL BEGINNING

Written August, 2014
*This piece was written as part of an ongoing training program that I
produced for a remote strength & conditioning client, who
was also a Jiu-Jitsu practitioner.*

I think of people's progress in Jiu-Jitsu as a progress through
certain conceptual stages. Simply put, you think of Jiu-Jitsu different-
ly as you progress through the ranks (or ideally, you progress
through the ranks because your understanding changes). If you had
the chance to look at the original curriculum I designed for my students at The Fight Gym, then you already have a bit of an idea of
what I'm talking about. In the beginning the curriculum is very con-
crete, but as the belt level gets higher the curriculum material gets
more vague: a blue belt may have to know these or those 6 techniques, but a purple belt has to show effective chain attacks, combin-
ing the threat of submission with sweep or transition attempts. The
idea here is to "test" how the student is "seeing" the situations as
they occur. Is he starting to organize information in his mind such
that he is able to recognize when certain conditions offer opportunities either for a submission or a transition, etc.? Is he thinking about
what is happening the way a _____ belt thinks about what is happening?

When we're new to Jiu-Jitsu, we learn that the joints of the human body have limitations: that when they're pushed beyond a certain point they will sustain damage. This is a blue or an early purple belt's understanding: there are positions, and within those positions arms and legs go all over the place, and maybe an arm or a leg gets toward an extreme, and I can make it go farther into the extreme.

I think a lot of people—I might even say most people—stay in this concept of Jiu-Jitsu forever. I hold the guy until I can set up my submission, then I execute. Guys get very sharp at this sort of game, and are able to tap a lot of people, and accordingly they are often satisfied to spend more and more time sharpening this sword, living within this concept (and patting themselves on the back for how good they are, judging by how many people they beat). Often they are awarded belts for doing so.

There is nothing really wrong with this, so long as the person in question enjoys what he or she is doing, and can do it without sustaining injury, etc. It is, however, a rudimentary relationship to the material, and there is a conceptual stage beyond this that, as far as I'm concerned, is the real beginning of Jiu-Jitsu.

A lot of guys spend their time on the mat pursuing knowledge of Jiu-Jitsu as they would a foreign country. They learn its language, its customs, its rituals, etc. They delve further and further into it, looking further and further afield for knowledge and secrets. I am by no means a master, and I am certainly not a world champion, but I can say absolutely that my Jiu-Jitsu did not get decent until I stopped looking "out there" for answers and insights, until I realized that what Jiu-Jitsu was trying to show me was not a foreign country called Jiu-Jitsu but rather my own body (and, through my body, the body of every other human being with two arms and two legs and a heart and lungs...)

Once I realized this, the delineation between "position" and "submission" dissolved into the broader concept of leverage—not as a word we throw around on the mat in regard to this or that submis-

200

sion, but leverage as a manifestation of macro-level mechanical functionality (as a product of proper alignment) opposing macro-level mechanical failure or inefficiency (as a product of improper alignment) which, when considered in its earlier stages, we call positional advancement and control and which, in its later stages, we call submission.

Aren't both positional control and submission finally a question of moving my opponent's limbs into an unideal position? If effectiveness is a question of efficiency and orientation then by negating his effectiveness I am simultaneously moving his limb toward the margins of its functionality. And once it is moved outside its range of functionality, it is more easily moved into the further range, and further and further, until the true limitation of the joint (not simply muscular functionality) is compromised.

Since this is getting a little esoteric, let me give you an example. When my opponent is in my guard, he has to use his arms to maintain my distance from him (either my pulling him down or my sitting up into him). He is working to oppose my force primarily in two directions: forward and down. He therefore frames off my chest/torso. The most effective (efficient and functional) way for him to do this is with a straight (elbow locked) arm (or two arms), engaged at a 45-degree angle with my torso. This frame bears the force I will attempt to create with my pull, and does so effectively and efficiently. From here he can maintain his posture (and thus his control over his own body) and start to plot his own course.

Now, consider a common but far less efficient variation. He frames on my torso, but he does so with his elbows bent (and maybe slightly flared). This is a weaker frame, but he is able to oppose my pull for some time, until the force overwhelms his muscular endurance. Now, let's say I begin to pull on his elbow, moving his arm into a less and less effective (efficient/functional) position. At a certain point, the effectiveness value of his push falls below the effectiveness value of my pull; the arm ceases to bear weight, and my opponent collapses forward. What if now we continue to exploit the situation, and force the arm further along the same track? Soon the situation is no longer a question of moving outside the effective parameters of the limb's orientation to me, but outside the true functional parameters of the limb itself, i.e. forcing the shoulder joint beyond its mechanical limitation (in this case by applying a Kimura or omoplata shoulder lock).

Obviously the set-up is one with which any blue belt is familiar: break the guy down and shoulder lock him. Even the specific execution—open his elbow when you break him down so that you can move naturally into the Kimura—is far from "advanced." However, the perspective—to see submission as the furthest manifestation of a leverage disparity that began much earlier, that manifested first as effective positioning, then as positional advancement (breaking the guy down) and finally as a submission (the Kimura)—is, I think, something different.

I've talked previously about physical effectiveness as a function of proper alignment, of orienting myself to physical demand in the safest and most effective way possible. I've spent a good deal of time talking about it in terms of defense. Now, turn it around. When my opponent is not in proper position, what are the flaws in his position—the cracks in the dam that, with the force of the water behind them, become bigger and bigger until the whole thing fails?

Effective Jiu-Jitsu is about seeing the limitations of my own body as a blueprint for my opponents' bodies: not simply as a question of submission, but as a question of his macro-level ability to oppose me, to create an effect within our exchange. Any leverage discrepancy, taken to its furthest limit, is a submission: it moves a limb from its effective alignment into its ineffective alignment into the end of its mechanical range. Impose a limitation on a limb, force it to work outside its normal range, and continue to impose that pressure (effectively reducing his ability to oppose it with each incremental advancement) until we reach the true limit. Here, he can only tap.

OLD MAN JIU-JITSU

Written August, 2014
*This piece was written as part of an ongoing training program that I
produced for a remote strength & conditioning client, who
was also a Jiu-Jitsu practitioner.*

"My goal is never to win. My goal is don't get defeat."

—Master Rickson Gracie

Let's face it: we're not getting any younger, and nowhere will that
be more apparent than on the mat. The "fire" and "vigor" of youth—
the readiness of energy, and the willingness to expend it as though it
is and always will be in limitless supply—begins to wane, and we find
ourselves outpaced (note: I didn't say outmatched) by young and
eager lower belts. We find ourselves surprised by how much energy
our younger opponent is willing to give a technique that, on its merits, shouldn't work, and may even find ourselves surprised
(annoyed?) when, seemingly by virtue of his tenacity alone, that
technique succeeds (or at least gets farther along than it should). We
find ourselves losing scrambles and failing at sweeps due to our opponents' athletic and borderline gymnastic maneuvering. We have to
fight—really fight—to open their guard, escape their back control,

203

etc., simply because they will not give up on a grip or a position whose viability has expired.

Such is the nature of grappling. One of the biggest misconceptions I see tossed around the BJJ community is the idea that, because technique can beat size and strength, size and strength don't (or shouldn't) matter. In fact, Jiu-Jitsu exists precisely because size and strength do matter, and they matter A LOT (and Helio would have been the first one to say this). Understanding this means also understanding that, just because something isn't technical Jiu-Jitsu, that does not mean it can't hurt me (just as, just because I can use a technique to hurt someone, that doesn't mean it's Jiu-Jitsu). I think of the headlock as the epitome of this situation: the headlock is not a technical choke (it doesn't make very clean contact with either the carotids or the trachea), is not an efficient means of control (I am holding my opponent by literally holding him in place, not by compromising his maneuverability), and offers little to no opportunity for advancement (if I am in a side headlock and I let go of the headlock to try to take mount or knee-on-belly, I will very likely lose everything when I create the necessary disconnection from my opponent). AND YET: if you've ever been underneath someone fully committed to holding you in a headlock, you know that the headlock can be an absolute bear to escape.

So: should our understanding that the headlock can be problematic, that it can possibly even result in a crude choke or a neck crank, lead us to the conclusion that we should attempt to apply the headlock? Certainly not: we understand the qualities of the headlock versus the qualities of other options in the same situations; we can ascribe a value to that strategy, when compared to other strategies. The cons outweigh the pros, while the pros for establishing a technical side control outweigh the cons. Obviously, there's no contest here. Being the old man on the mat means understanding the difference between something's ability to hurt me and it's adherence to the Jiu-Jitsu criteria (can I do this efficiently? can I do this while maintaining my own safety?), about knowing where the line is in everything, and pursuing technically sound Jiu-Jitsu while defending everything, technical or not.

The headlock situation is obvious, but consider another situation: We accept the down position against a strong young white belt who has a wrestling background. The wrestler stands and approaches with his arms extended to grip our pants, then releases the pants as he scrambles to north-south. He arrives there with no control of our arms, legs, or head, but is heavy and tight. I can choose to make my first move at any point in this progress, so at what point do I decide to engage?

1) I engage early, while he is still standing, and attempt to make contact with his collar or leg. What sort of a response should I expect? Most likely the wrestler will explosively disengage, then change the angle and reengage in an attempt to pass my guard. If I attempt to thwart those efforts, I will likely end up in a scramble in which I may succeed in neutralizing his efforts, I may fight my way to top position, or my opponent's favorable mobility (he's already on his feet or knees) may determine the course of the coming moments.

2) I wait until he passes, protect the handles (the points on my body he would use to flatten me, my face, elbow, and knee), and then engage with my frames, using my skeleton to efficiently bear his pressure. I work to recover now that he is close and has stopped moving in an unpredictable and rapid fashion. If he disengages from my frames, I either recover or, if he turns the corner, again defend the handles, allowing him to do all the work of running. Eventually, due to his inability to immobilize me (by my proper application of defensive mindset) I recover to a control position, and can now begin to mechanically impair him to the point of submission.

Which approach is right? Both are. Both fall within the margins of what could be called Jiu-Jitsu, and moreover: both can be successfully employed. The question is, then: Which should *I* do? If I know that my opponent is willing to give an inordinate amount of energy to a scramble—either because he is young and full of energy, or because he doesn't know any better—then it is somewhat foolish to attempt to implement a scramble-dependent strategy. I know that path is going to be hard, and very likely I am at best going to recover guard: why not wait until he has made contact—and stopped running around like crazy—to pursue the same goal?

So we arrive at the key delineation for the aging (I didn't say old, I said aging) grappler: the delineation between what I can do based on my personal level of strength, fitness, athleticism, body aware- ness, and willingness to expend energy, and what I can do when those things are either stripped away or else inferior when compared to those possessed by my opponent. This is, of course, THE question in BJJ, and yet—despite the lip service paid to "being technical," "not using strength," etc.—I think this consideration all too often falls by the wayside, particularly in competition-oriented schools, in which it is possible to basically guarantee size and strength similarity between a student and his or her potential opponent, and to condition for a particular moment in time, i.e. the day of the tournament.

Obviously it is fun to be athletic, to get into those epic death matches, to clash against an opponent using all of your strength and fortitude and tenacity, to leave it all on the mat. This is, however, not the true aim of the art. The real question is always: What can I make work, when I have no physical advantage? What core techniques, strategies, and concepts remain, when I take away what "I" can do? As we age, as we understand ourselves as owning limited reserves of energy, as we become cynical about the meaning or value of these gym wars, this is the question that we confront. So ask yourself, when you're on the mat: Is what I'm doing a "headlock"? Is it some- thing that is only working because of my willingness to put excess strength and energy into it? It can be enjoyable to use Jiu-Jitsu as a sword—to go out and impose and dominate and smash—but this should never make us lose sight of the fact that Jiu-Jitsu was always meant to be a shield. A lot of guys who "age out" of their ability to use Jiu-Jitsu as a sword never make the mental switch: they keep trying to "fight" with the young guns. At a certain point, this just isn't a realistic goal. A change to a defensive mindset becomes necessary for us to stay on the mats and, more than that, to actually enjoy that time. My goal is to enjoy what my body can do now while it can still do it, but to understand (as best I can) what among those attributes will fade, and to lay the foundation of my Jiu-Jitsu on a core of techniques and a style and a mentality that will serve me long after I've aged out of my physical prime.

DO HOLD YOUR BREATH

Written October, 2014
This piece was written as part of an ongoing training
program I produced for a private client.

This is something I've been working on lately, and that I've found very useful in my Jiu-Jitsu (and my life in general), both physically and mentally. That being said, it does take a fair amount of time and energy, and it can be fairly unpleasant. I'm sharing it because I think it's valuable, but I also understand that it's not everyone's cup of tea.

Being able to hold your breath for a long period of time isn't, for me at least, really about holding the breath at all. I've talked before about the distance between Fear (the physiological response to perceived threat or danger) and the Event (the actual occurrence, in real time, of the event that Fear was warning us about), but to reiterate (or maybe just to restate): I am going through my life, living in the present but aware of/"predicting" the future (I'm aware of things that are headed my way, whether it's a truck in the road ahead or a big job interview I have on Monday); I perceive, in the amorphous realm of the potential futures my brain is always imagining, a threat to my health/wellbeing/social status/etc.; I experience stress (physical, mental, emotional); my heart rate is elevated; I become inclined toward militant and defensive

208

thoughts (I feel like I am literally "under attack"); my focus is drawn further into the potential future, leaving less and less awareness of the present moment; etc., etc. In short, Fear (which, remember is NOT the Event, merely the imagining of the Event) can literally change my experience of the world, change my outlook, change my personality (I think you've probably met, as I have, people who become habitually fearful, who relate to the world exclusively in this fashion, imagining always and only the dangers to be avoided).

If this were Fear's only sin, it would be a forgivable one (and we certainly cannot discount Fear's absolutely essential—you might even say singularly essential—role in man's survival as a species). However, Fear does not stop here. Fear makes a promise: the promise that it holds the key to eternal freedom from disaster, horror, and death. "Don't use your other modes of relating to the world," Fear says, "Don't stop and smell the flowers. Instead, think about the flowers' pollen! What if you have an undiscovered allergy? Better to stick with me and think ahead, I'll keep you safe...."

Fear seduces us with this promise, cordoning us into smaller and smaller rooms, always warning of the potential dangers just outside, like a well-intentioned but grossly overbearing mother. And, like an overbearing mother, Fear would always rather have you just stay inside—somewhere where she can "keep an eye on you"—than let you out into the wide, dangerous world.

Holding the breath is about how you live in the Fear: how you conduct yourself within the time when the Fear has begun to insist that it has something to tell you, something that you absolutely need to know and pay attention to and base your decisions on *right now*. It is about training yourself to manage your own emotional response, about choosing to conduct yourself with discretion and intelligence when the Fear wants you to freak out, flee, abort the mission, run for the hills. It is about everything Jiu-Jitsu is about, only more so, because here the Fear is very, very real. Because after all: you really do need to breathe.

More than even this, however, it is about acquainting yourself with a true danger (and I don't mean this in the thrill-seeking, adrenaline junkie way it sounds). It is about calibrating your Fear response to an essential stimulus, in the face of all of the manufactured Fear we are constantly bombarded with (Isis! Falling stock market! Less-than-hopeful holiday sales projections! Buy this body spray and drink this beer, or else everyone will think you're a loser and the hot girl won't talk to you!). We live in an environment of manufactured fear and, barring any actual experience by which to calibrate the veracity of these claims (how often does the average person encounter an actual threat?), our delicate (and highly adaptive) sensory apparatus calibrates itself to these signals: the TV tells me that this is a fearful thing, and so it must be! We're told that the threat is right outside the door, and so our thoughts go to fearful things when we step outside the door.

Fear is very clever. It will invent scenarios and then mine details from the environment, cherry-picking some and discarding others to paint a more fearful picture than the facts present. It will laud its host for his or her "responsibility," his or her "level-headedness," for "thinking it through," and not being one of those people who "just rushes in." And, like the ambitious advisor to the impressionable king, it will impose itself further and further until the host is merely its puppet.

Am I promoting thoughtlessness? Am I suggesting that we abolish fear? Certainly not. I am suggesting that, by holding the breath, we reacquaint ourselves with Fear's true trustworthiness. We remind ourselves on the most primal, basic level that the Fear is not the Event itself.

It is worth noting, at this point, that extensive research has been done in this field, and that it is completely safe to practice (the holding itself, discounting environmental dangers: passing out while standing or underwater can of course be hazardous to health). The "blackout reflex" occurs well in advance of any brain damage (that is, in fact, the purpose of the blackout reflex: to begin to conserve oxygen in order to preserve the brain in the event of a prolonged period without oxygen).

How to Hold Your Breath

Most of us take it for granted that the primary purpose of respiration is the inhalation of oxygen, but this is simply not the case. An equal, and potentially even more essential purpose is the ventilation of carbon dioxide. As it turns out, the body is far more sensitive to changes in carbon dioxide levels than it is to changes in oxygen levels. Think about it: have you ever held your breath for a long time, and then violently exhaled, feeling like your lungs are going to burst? Why would you feel the need to release pressure, if the more primary goal was inhalation? As it turns out, the feeling of pressure is the buildup of CO_2, and does not necessarily indicate anything about the level of O_2 in the blood. Similarly, have you ever tried to build up a fire or blow up a balloon, and become lightheaded? This lightheadedness is your body's response to a drop in CO_2, which you've been "flushing" out via your more-aggressive-than-normal exhaling.

Try it right now. Hold your breath, and notice how the tension starts to build across the chest. You want to exhale; your body wants that CO_2 out!

One method for increasing the duration of the breath hold is to prepare by hyperventilating: by dropping the level of CO_2 in your blood below its normal level, and thus gaining the time it takes your body to return to and then exceed its normal level as regular cellular respiration takes place. This method is very effective: I took my "best hold time" from 1:17 to over 3 minutes the first time I tried it. (A quick note: Since you are artificially suppressing the body's CO_2 level and thus delaying the onset of the "breathe right now!" signals, it is possible for the body's level of O_2 to fall below the level necessary to sustain consciousness without any real, clear warning. This is not so bad: it's like getting choked out in Jiu-Jitsu. You pass out, start breathing, and wake up feeling very peaceful. However, because of this, the method I am going to describe should not be used in FREE diving, i.e. don't do this underwater.)

There are two types of breathing you use for this method: deep breathing and purge breathing. The deep breathing is designed to oxygenate the blood and slow the heart rate; purge breathing is designed to drop the body's CO_2 levels.

Deep Breathing: I do a 4-count inhale, 4-count hold, and an 8-count exhale. I've found this to be a very calming and effective pattern, but it is certainly not the only one. When I inhale, I think about the first 2-count going into my stomach, and the second 2 going into my chest and shoulders. So 1,2, stomach is expanding, 3, chest is expanding, 4, shoulders are going up. The hold gives the air you inhaled a chance to drop its O_2 and pick up CO_2. The 8-count exhalation should be done with a slight tightness in the throat, so that the breath makes a hissing sound. This resistance is said to increase inter-thoracic pressure and force more O_2 into the bloodstream.

Purge Breathing: I do a 2-count inhale, a 1-count hold, and a 2-count exhale. I have used different methods for the exhale, including blowing like I'm trying to build up a fire, but my best time was done with what I'm calling the "deep sigh" method: I exhale from the back of the throat with the mouth open wide like a funnel, like I had onions for lunch and I want to show someone how bad my breath is. I make an audible sigh when I do this which, although it sounds a little bit weird to anyone listening from the next room, is said to have a calming effect on the entire nervous system (think of how calm you feel after a deep yawn).

Method 1

This is the first way I tried. Sit or lay comfortably. Try to hold yourself in such a way that you don't have to hold any tension in your body at all. Tension is muscular work, which uses up O_2 and produces CO_2.

Breathe up and first hold:

90 seconds deep breathing
75 seconds purge breathing
90-second hold (only hold this long, even if you feel like you can go longer)
3-5 purge breaths, to release all of the accumulated CO_2

Breathe up and second hold:

90 seconds deep breathing
90 seconds purge breathing
150-second (2.5 min) hold (again, only hold this long, even if you feel like you can go longer)
3-5 purge breaths

Breathe up and third hold:

120 seconds deep breathing
105 seconds purge breathing
Hold for as long as you can.
3-10 purge breaths (until normal breathing can be restored).

Method 2

This is the method that I've been practicing lately. This method is a simple ladder, comprised of equal intervals of breathing and holding. Again, find a comfortable position.

Breathe up and first hold:

30 seconds deep breathing
30 seconds purge breathing
60-second hold

Breathe up and second hold:
60 seconds deep breathing
60 seconds purge breathing
120-second hold

Breathe up and third hold:

90 seconds deep breathing
90 seconds purge breathing
180-second hold

...and so on, increasing the breathing phases by 30 seconds and the holding phase by 60 seconds each time until you can no longer match the hold time to the breath time.

Method 3

Method 3 is the true hold, i.e. the little-to-no prep hold. This is not the method by which I have achieved my best time (or anything close to it), but it is in some ways the more rewarding. Since I began training with the first two methods, I've increased my little-to-no prep hold time by more than 45 seconds: in part, I'm sure, due to physiological changes, but in large part due to my familiarity with the signals and the accompanying Fear, and my increasing ability to maintain my composure throughout. Method 3 is, in some ways, the "proving ground" for the first two methods: the place you come to test what you've learned by practicing them.

6 deep breaths

6 purge breaths
Hold as long as you can.

Repeat until your hold time stops increasing.

I hope that you found all of that interesting. I can honestly say that, when I decided that I wanted to start trying to increase my breath holding ability, I vaguely expected a certain amount of carryover to other physical endeavors. While I certainly have found that to be the case, the practice has been far more rewarding, and in more ways, than I could have ever guessed it would be.

ATEMI WAZA

This piece was written in September, 2016,
as preparation work for a seminar I was scheduled to teach.
It is previously unpublished.

"Nothing is barred when it comes to protecting yourself against the attack of a vicious man."

— Martin "Farmer" Burns

For a variety of reasons, in recent years, a division has formed between those who profess that Gracie Jiu-Jitsu is a complete martial art on its own, and those who feel that a practitioner needs to supplement his or her Jiu-Jitsu with tools from other styles (i.e. striking styles) for that practitioner to have a "well-rounded" skill set.

From where I'm standing, a lot of these disagreements arise from misunderstandings on both sides. Often times you hear proponents of Gracie Jiu-Jitsu draw a hard line and say that only a grappling-only style represents "true" Jiu-Jitsu: that any incorporation of striking is a philosophical betrayal of the art, and as a strategy is mutually exclusive with the strategy of Gracie Jiu-Jitsu. On the other side, proponents of the "supplement-with-other skills" approach point to MMA as evidence that strikers do well in real fights all the time: that the

Gracies' assessment that "striking is a low-percentage strategy" is not reflected in the evidence and amounts to just so much marketing.

So, a few points to consider:

First, MMA is an excellent venue—and the hours and hours of recorded fights that we now have access to is an excellent resource—for determining what "works" in a real fight situation. However, as is often pointed out by the Gracies, the sport of modern MMA includes a few parameters that keep it from being a true one-to-one indicator for no-rules or "street" fighting. For one thing, the vast majority of modern MMA fights are weight class fights. This means that the fighters enjoy the luxury of knowing that the person they face will never be too much bigger than them. This may seem like a small point, but it goes a long way to determining the likelihood of the success of a striking strategy. Trading blows with someone my own size, more or less, is a vastly different undertaking from trading blows with someone much bigger, heavier, and likely stronger than myself. Under these conditions, "standing in the pocket" pales in comparison to the "too far to be hit or too close to be hurt" approach that forms the base of the Gracie strategy.

Second, striking in MMA, to a large extent, means striking with closed fists, an approach that becomes problematic in the absence of taped hands and gloves. As is often pointed out, gloves serve primarily to protect the hands of the one throwing the strikes, not the brain of the one receiving them. Without these protective measures, the hands prove to be much more problematic weapons.

Third—and this is a point often made by the Gracies—striking from the feet is a fundamentally unreliable strategy. This point explains itself when we consider the difference between striking an opponent when we are both standing, and striking an opponent when I have him mounted. Clearly the latter situation—in which my opponent is essentially held in place—gives me a far better vantage from which to land successful blows. From the feet, the specific combination of strike, angle, force, target orientation, etc., required to deliver a fight-ending strike, while not impossible, is certainly much harder to achieve. Or imagine it this way: if my intention is to knock my opponent unconscious, do I have a greater chance of doing this while standing facing him, while he is free to move closer and farther, bob and weave, etc., not to mention strike back at me with equal if not greater (if he is bigger) force, or would this same objective be more reliably achieved by essentially running into him, dragging him to the ground, and achieving a top position from which I am able to deliver powerful strikes but my opponent is not?

I often tell my classes that there are no good or bad tools: that true skill lies in knowing what a given tool is and is not good for. A headlock, for example, is a solid method for controlling someone and a passable means of choking them; understanding this means being able to make a better decision about how much I can reasonably expect to accomplish, should I manage to get my opponent in a headlock. How much energy do I expend holding my opponent, and how much do I expend in attempting to choke him? The ability to make these determinations is, in essence, the ability to manage my energy, and put it to its best use: in other words, the necessary skill for working efficiently, the core priority of Gracie Jiu-Jitsu, and an absolute essential should I find myself in a fight with a bigger, stronger opponent.

Which brings me to the point of this post, which is simply this: strikes are neither good tools nor bad tools; they, like all tools, have ideal uses and specific capabilities (and limitations), and when applied with this understanding can be fantastically effective. Throwing a right cross in an attempt to knock my opponent out may provide mixed results, given the combination of factors that must occur for a successful knockout blow, but throwing a right cross to get my opponent to cover his face and head with his arms—so that his legs are exposed for a takedown—is very reliable and very achievable.

Which brings me to a further point: The ideological division that exists now between some schools of thought is a false one, because

Kodokan Judo—the art that Maeda taught to the Gracies—incorporated striking. Even modern Judo, if one can find a traditional program, teaches *atemi waza*—striking techniques. The question is and always has been: To what end are the strikes being employed? If they are employed as a means unto themselves—I hit my opponent and he is incapacitated—they remain a fundamentally unreliable methodology. But when employed in service of an overall strategy of progressive positional control and submission, they can become a powerful and reliable tool.

This post is not meant to advocate "smash-jitsu," or the use of strikes in place of nuanced understanding and manipulation of an opponent. This post is simply to say that these tribal divisions that I see growing between MMA grapplers and traditional Gracie Jiu-Jitsu fighters does a disservice to both groups. Gracie Jiu-Jitsu is a complete martial art for MMA, self defense, etc., but only when the whole of the art is embraced, understood, and taught. I therefore encourage all practitioners to familiarize themselves with the techniques and strategies of *atemi waza*.

YOUR LOVE MEANS NOTHING

Written January, 2017. Previously unpublished

Sometimes, training goes well. We find ourselves having more success on the mat; we feel like things are falling into place for us mentally; we feel capable and confident in our emerging abilities.

Other times, training does not go well. For days (or weeks, or months) we feel like nothing is working, like nothing makes sense, like everything that was easy has become hard and everything that felt natural has become unnatural again.

What's worse, during these times, we may feel unsure about how to get ourselves back on track. Somehow we lost "it," and we're not sure what to do to get "it" back.

Students in this latter situation often approach me for advice. Some of the ideas I share with them are included below. The main point of this post will follow afterwards.

Assess your rolls, and take notes.

If you're anything like me, you spend a significant amount of time after training thinking about training: what worked, what didn't, what you tried, etc. Take a moment and put pen to paper. Make a few notes. Identify *in writing* situations in which you felt uncomfortable or insecure. Then, make these situations your personal project. I know what you're going to say: But coach, I need to work on everything! I know. So do I. But everything is not a thing. Yes, you need to get better at everything, but everything has to start with something. Pick a thing to work on, and work on that situation intentionally during your next training sessions. If you do not see solutions to the problems you're having, ask questions. Be willing to spend weeks working on a single situation or a handful of situations during open mat.

Make knowledge your goal.

I've said it before: Success is not the goal. Refinement is the goal. Success is the product of refinement. The gym is not a Roman colosseum. It is a workshop where we refine our craft. I'll try to make beautiful, clean, efficient, controlled Jiu-Jitsu, and you try to do the same. In this, we can both succeed. Success in this does not require some of us to fail and some of us to succeed; in this everyone in the room can succeed at the same time! If instead I am trying only to make victories, my success is defined by someone else's loss. I feel increased, the other person feels diminished, the net remains the same. I mention this because often a student's feeling that he has lost "it" stems from his sense that now he is unable to perform as well against his peers. The sense that he has been in some way diminished comes from the loss of his previous feeling of increase. Remember that true progression does not come at the expense of vanquished training partners, nor does my training partner's success mean that I am less. Another thing you've heard me say if you've ever trained with me: The biggest winner is the guy who learns the most. He goes home with the biggest prize.

Work defense.

I'm not the first person to say this, but it's worth saying again: Gracie Jiu-Jitsu is a self-defense art. If you can't keep yourself safe, then you may not survive long enough to win. When things go sideways and you're feeling overmatched, strong self-defense from every position is the solid footing that stops you from sliding all the way down the mountain to your grisly demise. You simply cannot be too good at, or have too much practice implementing, the self-defense core of the art. You just can't. From this perspective someone mounting you is no longer a devastating blow to your morale, but rather a welcome opportunity to improve a vital skill set (a skill set which, during your reign as a one man offensive terror, you likely never had to develop).

In my experience, these preceding points are very effective methods for overcoming lulls in your progression. However, there is a more essential point that sometimes goes unmentioned when this subject comes up.

I know you love Jiu-Jitsu. I see it on your social media pages. I see you repping the latest gi from the newest company. I see you #bjjlifestyle-ing everything. I'm not questioning your love. What I am saying is: So what? So you love Jiu-Jitsu. So f*cking what?

Improvement in Jiu-Jitsu requires one thing over everything else: time on the mat. Jiu-Jitsu has to soak into your body. It has to rewire your thinking. You have to develop motor skills and neural pathways that you didn't have before, and that takes time. When students approach me and ask what they can do to improve their Jiu-Jitsu, the question I usually ask in reply is: How much is Jiu-Jitsu a priority for you? How many hours do you give Jiu-Jitsu in a given week?

I ask this question because often there is a serious disconnect between the amount of time a student *feels* they are involved in Jiu-Jitsu and the amount of time they actually spend training (and yes, I understand that thinking about Jiu-Jitsu while off the mat does have a place in learning and progress. That falls into the same category as journalling your rolls, mentioned above. I'm not talking about that). If, in an average week, you spend literally 3-4 hours training (say 2 classes of 2 hrs each, or 2 1-hour classes and an open mat) then that is the true marker of how highly you prioritize Jiu-Jitsu.

The question to ask, then, is: By this metric, what do you prioritize more highly than Jiu-Jitsu? Many of you probably spend more than four hours a week watching football. Or sitting in traffic. Or shopping for groceries. Or googling yourself.

Now, the important thing to realize about this is: This is not a judgement. This is simply a tool for recognizing our own behavior, for seeing ourselves honestly, not as we would like to be. If you prioritize spending time with your kids, or working so you can buy a house, or working on your car, I am not saying you are doing the wrong thing. I am saying: Expect to make progress in the areas and on the things you have prioritized, and don't be surprised when the things you have de-prioritized languish.

Hence the title of this post. Your love of Jiu-Jitsu means absolutely nothing, when it comes to your skill level, if your love does not manifest itself in you making the time. And, like most things with Jiu-Jitsu, what is true of the art is true of everything else. In the current cultural climate, I encourage everyone to remember that caring is not enough. Caring, without action, is literally worth nothing. It makes nothing. It changes nothing. It is nothing. Put your time where your heart is, and I promise that you'll see growth there.

MEDITATE ON ONENESS

Written July 27, 2015. Previously unpublished.

When you train BJJ, you find yourself pondering possibilities.

How can I sweep someone from this position? How can I achieve an arm lock from here or there? How can I sink in this choke, or hit that pass?

We are, in effect, pondering the nature and character of our opponents' inherent anatomical weakness, asking essentially: Under what conditions can an elbow or a shoulder joint be made to transgress the limits of its functionality? Under what conditions does the brain shut off?

When we ponder these things, we ponder the nature and character of the human mechanism itself. We are meditating on the nature of the body and its capabilities, its strengths and weaknesses.

It seems to me that for many people, BJJ never becomes anything more than this. It remains forever the shallow consideration of base mechanics, a means to an end, a crass and militant method for inflicting violence and damage upon another person.

Certainly, it is that. It is a fighting art, a self-defense art. It is the study of inflicting pain and damage. But if it remains this, it will always be less than it might be.

224

I fear that, for many people, BJJ feeds a forgivable but no less objectionable delusion. As humans we tend to make deals with life, bargains with God. Someone dies and we ask, "What happened?" We hear the answer, and are relieved that we do not do whatever that person did, and are therefore immune to their manner of death. ("He had a heart attack? I'm in better shape than he was!" "Car accident? I'm a more careful driver than he was!" "Lung cancer? I'm not a smoker!")

It is certainly a forgivable comfort to seek, but its forgivability makes it no more legitimate. Of course death in all its many forms finds everyone, regardless of the deals we imagine we've made with life. Such delusions comprise nothing, finally, but a lie we tell ourselves, often with subtle but no less unsettling consequences.

Because to ascribe culpability to the deceased is to declare our difference from them. He was A... Thank God that I'm B, and am therefore unlike him! But of course every death is the same: the human machine has surpassed its furthest tolerance. And in that we are all alike: we inhabit bodies which require a fairly narrow set of conditions to endure. Raise or lower its internal temperature ten degrees, turn its head a few degrees more, expose its brain to a force beyond a given threshold, and the result is the same: the limit is reached, and death is achieved. The delusion that such cannot happen to you as well—that you by your very being are somehow fundamentally far from if not immune to such extremes—is just that: a delusion.

Again, I fear that too many people relate to BJJ in this way. Somewhere deep in their hearts they believe that if they get good enough, they will somehow become immune to the weaknesses of the flesh. They gleefully choke others' necks and lock others' joints, convincing themselves with each submission that they are essentially something different from their victim: that such weakness or vulnerability has been evicted from their being; that they are something Other and immune.

The opposite, though true, is harder to consider. It is more unsettling to see in another's weakness your own weakness: harder to see in another's vulnerability your own vulnerability. It is less comforting to consider the notion that, despite your years of training, you are made of the same stuff you were made of in the beginning, that you live in an essentially weak and breakable machine, one which should be regarded with care. And this, to me, is exactly the source of BJJ's greatest offering: that you begin to comprehend all of humanity as one entity, made uniform by our limitation and weakness, and thus deserving always of our compassion and mercy. Because there is no lasting strength. There is no deal with God. We are all, each of us, a small and naked creature set upon a world full of forces much greater than ourselves: a world capable of horrors beyond our limited comprehension.

This, to me, is the heart of Jiu-Jitsu: that we are all the same. That we must be kind to one another—we must be merciful—because we are small and limited and weak, and because nothing else in this universe will be kind or merciful.

Strength fades. Meditate on your weakness, your smallness. These things are the truth of you. These are what Jiu-Jitsu is here to reveal to you. All else is vanity and delusion and fear. One day the world will overcome you. One day your furthest limit will be surpassed, and you will disappear into the void. While you are here, meditate on mercy. In the end, it really is all we have to offer one another.

BLUE CORNER

Written November 17, 2009. This piece was written on spec for a popular literary magazine that was doing an issue on MMA. It is previously unpublished.

The floor manager calls our names off a clipboard. There are only two guys missing, and neither of them is the guy I'm fighting. The guy I'm fighting is sitting behind me, talking on my cornerman's cell phone.

"That's funny," says my cornerman, when the floor manager calls my opponent's name and the kid behind us raises his hand. "He just asked if he could use my phone. I guess his cornermen haven't shown up yet."

"That sucks for him," I say, raising my hand as the floor manager calls my name. The kid behind us looks me over, and then hands my cornerman's phone back.

"All right," says the floor manager. "Go down to the locker room and get your physicals."

We all shuffle past the cage, up the stairs onto the venue's stage, and then through a doorway and down a set of stairs to the cinderblock locker room. The doctors are set up on either side of a long card table, wearing latex gloves and holding stethoscopes. A skinny kid wearing a tee-shirt with the logo of the fight promotion on the breast pocket hands out sheets for us to fill out. Nobody has a pen. Someone finds one, and we wait while it gets passed around. The doctors speak in hushed tones to the fighters they are checking. No one else is talking.

"When the doctor asks me if I've had any concussions," says the guy waiting in front of me in line, "I'm just going to say, 'None that I can remember.' That way I don't have to lie to him."

"I'm not sure you have to worry about it," I say. The physical doesn't seem all that involved. Everybody has been in and out of the doctor's chair in less than two minutes. The line is moving pretty quickly, anyway. The floor manager comes in through the exit carrying a box.

"When I call your name," he says, "come and get your gloves."

"You fought before?" asks the concussion kid.

"No," I say. "Have you?"

"Just once."

"How'd it go?"

"I got knocked the fuck out," he says, laughing. "I woke up in the locker room."

"Jesus," I say.

"Don't matter," he says. "I just want to fight."

The line moves another step forward. I look at the two guys leaving the doctor's chairs. One of them yawns. He checks his watch. The kid I'm fighting is in line to see the other doctor, a couple feet ahead of me. I stare at the back of his head. Then the floor manager calls my name. I raise my hand and he comes over to me.

"What are you," he says, "a large?"

"I guess," I say. I hold up my hands.

He nods. "Blue corner?" he asks.

"Blue corner," I say.

I take the gloves he hands me. I look them over.

"These gloves have blood on them," I say.

"They all do," he says. "Don't worry about it. Who are you fighting?"

I point to the kid in the other line. The kid is looking back at us.

"Here," says the floor manager. He throws the kid a pair of red gloves. "If those don't fit, come find me."

The kid and I exchange nods, and then look forward again. The lines are still moving. Captain Concussion sits down. I hear the doctor ask him if he's had any concussions and I see him shake his head. Has he ever been knocked out? Once, he admits, in his last fight. And how long ago was that? Two months. The doctor checks his blood pressure. Someone hands me the pen that's being passed around. On the other side of the table, the doctor signs off on my opponent's medical sheet. The fighters who were checked off first are changing out of their street clothes.

There's still almost an hour until the first bell, but the noise from upstairs is already getting louder. I look at the blood dried on the gloves in my hands. Then the doctor calls for the next person. I sit down facing the rest of the line. After me is a huge middle-eastern-looking man with "Brown Pride" tattooed sloppily across his upper chest. The doctor asks if I've ever had a concussion, ever been knocked out, if I have any known medical problems. He asks me how many times I've fought before. I tell him this is my first fight. He checks my blood pressure and listens to my heart. He wishes me good luck, and signs my sheet.

My cornerman is waiting for me in the other locker room, the locker room for the blue corner. He hands me the bag holding my shorts and cup and mouthpiece. I show him the gloves they gave me.

"These still have blood on them," he says.

"I know," I say. "They told me not to worry about it."

He hands them back. "What do you want to do now?" he says.

"I don't know," I say. "What do you think I should do?"

"I don't know," he says. "Start warming up, I guess."

"How long until I fight?" I ask.

"At least an hour," he says. "On second thought, don't warm up yet."

We sit down and wait. There are a dozen other fighters in the room with us, plus their cornermen. Two guys set up a folding mat in one corner and start working escapes. In the corner opposite, another fighter is sleeping. One of the trainers starts taping hands. The referee comes in and goes over the rules. I wonder what the kid I'm set to fight is doing. I wonder if he's warming up. If he's warming up maybe I want to be warming up. Maybe if he's doing nothing I want to be warming up anyway. I tell my cornerman I'm going to start warming up.

"Ok," he says. "If that's what you feel like doing."

I go find a bathroom and change into my shorts. I wonder if I should try to pee now, because I don't want to have to go when it's time for me to fight. I remember being in the Christmas pageant back in fifth grade, and having to pee right as the teacher was getting us set up backstage. I try, but I don't really have to. I go back into the locker room and find my cornerman. I sit facing him while he tapes my hands.

"Keep your hands up," he says while he works. "Hack his legs. He's not going to like it. If he takes you down, don't worry about it. You know what to do. There's no way this kid's in better shape than you are. When you've got him hurt just let your hands go. Keep the pressure on him and he'll gas. Just keep your cool and stay safe. How does that feel?"

I work my hand open and closed. I've never had my hands taped before. I don't know what it's supposed to feel like.

"Fine," I say. "Or, I don't know. Kind of tight."

"Bad tight?" he says.

"No," I say, "I think it's all right."

He tapes the other hand. Then we put my gloves on, and I start warming up. My cornerman holds the big pad and I move with him and throw kicks. People are watching me, and I have no idea what they're thinking. I decide to think they're impressed and scared. I think maybe they're just annoyed at how much noise I'm making. I sit back down. I wonder again what my opponent is doing.

The floor manager comes in. He calls the first fighter's name, and says he should be on stage in five. The fighter's cornermen receive the information and relay it to the fighter, who is sitting two feet behind them. The fighter stands and starts shadowboxing, moving in a small circle, staring at the floor. Everybody's watching him without looking. Then the floor manager comes in and says it's time. The fighter and his cornermen go out. Everyone else crowds around the TV monitor. There's a delay in the feed. The noise from the crowd and the announcer upstairs comes out of sync with the action. The bell rings and the two come together in the middle of the ring. The fighter from our locker room throws a kick and loses his balance. The other fighter falls on top of him and starts punching. The referee steps in. I feel better, knowing that I can't look any worse than that. The floor manager sticks his head in and calls for the next fighter. He tells everyone to check the order and be up on stage as soon as their fight comes up. The next fighter leaves and the first one comes back, cursing and pulling off his gloves. He has a purple knot forming around one eye. Some of the others slap him on the back, offer sympathetic comments.

"It happens to the best of them," someone says.

"When am I up?" I say.

"You're the second after this one," says my cornerman. "Make sure you stay warm."

The next two fights go the distance. The fighters come back to the locker room looking battered and exhausted. One of them takes a bucket from his cornerman and throws up into it and then sits there holding it in both hands.

"We should probably get upstairs," says my cornerman.

We go up. My opponent and his cornerman are there on the other side of the stage. Down in the cage, the fight ends. The fighter from our corner connects with an overhand right that sends his opponent to the mat. We have to wait while the paramedics load the other fighter onto a backboard.

Then, the music starts. We walk to the edge. I tap my opponent on the shoulder, and when he turns I put out my hand and wish him good luck. He wishes me the same. Then the corridor leading from the stage stairs to the cage fills with dry ice fog, and the announcer calls his name. I watch him go. His cornerman is right behind him. Then the announcer calls my name. I walk out through the fog. Heavy metal is blaring through the speakers, but behind it I can hear people cheering. I stop on my mark, take off my shirt and my shoes. I grin to show the doctor my mouthpiece, knock on my cup to show him I'm wearing one. I close my eyes while he smears Vaseline across my brows and cheek bones. Then it's time. My cornerman hugs me. I climb the stairs and step inside.

"This is it," says the referee, as they close and latch the door. "Are you ready? Are you ready?"

My opponent and I just nod. We stare at each other across the empty cage between us, waiting for the bell to ring.

ABOUT THE AUTHOR

Scott Burr is a graduate of the creative writing program at The Colorado College. He is a black belt professor, first degree, in Brazilian Jiu-Jitsu. He is the first person to have earned the rank of black belt from American BJJ pioneer and sixth-degree black belt professor Steve Maxwell. To date, he is one of only three people to have earned the rank of black belt under Steve.

Scott also holds black belt rank in Kodokan Judo (shodan/first degree, awarded by representatives of the Konan Yudanshakai and certified by the Kodokan Judo Institute) and the Korean art of Kuk Sul Do (jo kyo/first degree, awarded and certified by Federation President and Grandmaster Choon Shik Yang).

Scott is a MaxwellSC-certified Pro Trainer, and holds Level 1 and Level 2 certifications in both the MaxwellSC Kettlebell and Bodyweight Training systems. He has appeared in many of Steve Maxwell's instructional videos as Steve's "designated demonstrator," and has traveled all over the world with Steve—from El Salvador to Croatia—assisting at seminars on everything from joint mobility to breathwork to kettlebell training to Brazilian Jiu-Jitsu.

Scott was the head BJJ instructor and strength & conditioning coach at The Fight Gym (originally an all-in-one MMA gym, and later a Brazilian Jiu-Jitsu school and strength & conditioning facility) for over a decade.

Scott is also the author of the strength & conditioning manuals *Suspend Your Disbelief: How to Build and Build Strength with the World's Most Rugged Suspension Training Device* and *Get a Grip: A Practical Primer on Grip Strength and Endurance… and More.*

Scott lives and teaches in Northeast Ohio.

www.ingramcontent.com/pod-product-compliance
Lightning Source LLC
Chambersburg PA
CBHW031153270326
41931CB00006B/253